"Anna Maria Bounds provides an imn
sis of the COVID-19 pandemic. It is o
demonstrates that, in 2020, Bounds w
at a terrible, terrible time. As it offer
spread throughout New York City, this
as a New Yorker, leading expertise on
thor, to provide a definitive account o
wider world's) history. To understand v
happened, how preppers readied for ar
be learned from these events, and how v
prepare for the next big event, you nee

"Anna Maria Bounds dives again into
this fascinating follow-up to her 2020 b
perience and ethnographic research of tl
bring an urgent update and focus on the
aster prepared in disastrous times. The s
conditions, governance, and racialized
puzzle that Anna brings to the table, in
of what is at stake. Expect fascinating s
man connection, energy for collective ac
learned during the pandemic that they cc
fall? Then read this book!"

M

"In her second book on the prepping con
captivating account of life in New York
peek inside the urban prepper movemer
hope, planning, and community can alla

URBAN PREPPERS AND THE PANDEMIC IN NEW YORK CITY

Drawing on urban and community resilience literature, *Urban Preppers and the Pandemic in New York City: Class, Resilience and Sheltering in Place* offers a detailed qualitative analysis of the impact of the COVID-19 pandemic on New York City and on the philosophy and practices of the city's urban prepper subculture.

With a special focus on the height of the pandemic in New York, this book considers the city's unique position as the pandemic's first epicenter in the United States. It also explores the lived experience of enduring the pandemic as reflections of class division, considering key themes, including the exodus of the wealthy, sheltering in place for the middle class, the inability to leave high-risk neighborhoods for the poor, and sheltering-in-place practices and community resilience efforts by New York preppers. It analyzes the importance of good government and an engaged citizenry in developing an agenda for the city's continued recovery and its future, underscoring the need for cities to develop disaster management approaches that expand traditional "command and control" models to make space for local knowledge and resources.

At its core, *Urban Preppers and the Pandemic in New York City: Class, Resilience and Sheltering in Place* is about understanding New York City's pandemic experience and how self-reliance evolves into community resilience outside of institutions. It is vital reading for scholars and students of sociology, anthropology, geography and urban studies with interests in subcultures, ethnography and the sociology of disasters.

Anna Maria Bounds is an Associate Professor of Sociology at Queens College, City University of New York, USA.

Routledge Studies in Urban Sociology

This series presents the latest research in urban sociology, welcoming both theoretical and empirical studies that focus on issues including urban conflict, politics and protest, social exclusion and social inclusion, urban regeneration and social class, and the ways in which these affect the social, economic, political, and cultural landscape of urban areas.

Titles in this series

Deindustrialization and Casinos
A Winning Hand?
Alissa Mazar

Urban Regeneration and Neoliberalism
The New Liverpool Home
Clare Kinsella

Entrepreneurial Governance in the Neoliberal Era
Local Government and the Automotive Industry
Oliver Cowart

Urban Preppers and the Pandemic in New York City
Class, Resilience and Sheltering in Place
Anna Maria Bounds

For more information about this series, please visit: www.routledge.com/sociology/series/RSUS

URBAN PREPPERS AND THE PANDEMIC IN NEW YORK CITY

Class, Resilience and Sheltering in Place

Anna Maria Bounds

Routledge
Taylor & Francis Group
LONDON AND NEW YORK

Designed cover image: Getty/GabrielPevide

First published 2025
by Routledge
4 Park Square, Milton Park, Abingdon, Oxon OX14 4RN

and by Routledge
605 Third Avenue, New York, NY 10158

Routledge is an imprint of the Taylor & Francis Group, an informa business

British Library Cataloguing-in-Publication Data
A catalogue record for this book is available from the British Library

ISBN: 978-1-032-50942-6 (hbk)
ISBN: 978-1-032-50944-0 (pbk)
ISBN: 978-1-003-40035-6 (ebk)

DOI: 10.4324/9781003400356

Typeset in Sabon
by Apex CoVantage, LLC

This book is dedicated to my beloved father,
Kenneth G. Schaffer, *the epitome of resiliency.*

In the U.S. Navy, my father earned the Vietnam Service medal, three Bronze Stars, the National Defense Medal and the Navy Achievement Medal. At home, he won the love and respect of all those who knew him, earning the titles of Husband, Father, Brother and Friend.

CONTENTS

ACKNOWLEDGMENTS

My sincere gratitude to the prepping community for sharing their insights and their pandemic experiences with me. Your willingness to share your knowledge and time to teach me preparedness skills has not just been generous; it has been a life saver.

I also share a deep appreciation for the many New Yorkers who discussed their pandemic experiences with me. Thank you to my Queens College students who have shared their resiliency and their positivity with me. My mind and my soul are richer for these gifts.

Thank you to Andy Beveridge for providing ongoing inspiration for my research. Through our conversations and his emails about a related article or event, he has always supported my work and he has always encouraged me when the chips were down. He is a real-life Obi Wan. Thank you to Robert Beauregard for providing invaluable guidance throughout my academic career. When I was in graduate school, he called my interests "quirky but important." He's still right. I am also grateful to Meg Holden for our friendship and for her intellectual fierceness. Since graduate school, Meg and I have spent our lives exploring quirky and meaningful ideas.

I am grateful to the gifted and generous group of colleagues dedicated to researching prepping subculture. My special thanks to Michael F. Mills, Bradley Garrett, Keiza Barker and Chris Ellis for their hard work in blazing the trail. Our intellectual exchanges and our support of one another are transforming an emerging field into a rich literature – "We few, We happy few, We band of [researchers]."

My heartfelt thanks are extended to Taylor & Francis and to my editor, Neil Jordan. Neil's insight and support have been immense. Peter Heap, the editor of my two books, is an intellectual force in my life. In another life, he is a famous philosopher on the lecture circuit. I read all of his essays and I write far too complicated letters to him. He responds with letters that offer deep insight and that raise even more interesting questions. John Emrich has been an outstanding research assistant. His attention to detail and quick responses have been amazing. Jo Barnett has also been a terrific assistant and an even more wonderful friend.

I am also especially grateful for the love of Susan and Liam; their brightness has guided our family from loss to happiness. I am also thankful to Rick, our family's best friend and neighbor, for providing encouragement after the loss of my father. For our ongoing conversations about our love for the city, many thanks to Asa, Christa, Sandy, Sue and Suzanne. As always, I am so grateful for those that I meet at the campfire.

Thank you, most of all, to my husband for his love, his sense of humor and his support.

1

PREPARING FOR SURVIVAL VERSUS TRYING TO SURVIVE

There has always been one thing that I have hated about being a New Yorker. It's not the noise, the traffic, the expense or the eight million other people. I can deal with all of those things – I love the city. I hate what you have to contend with when being introduced as a New Yorker. In the first moments of the conversation, you get to bask in the glory and celebrity of the city (Yes, it is that beautiful. Yes, it is that bold. Yes, it is that magical. And, yes, non-New Yorkers have the right to be envious of you). But before the imaginary soundtrack of Alicia Keyes and Jay-Z singing about your beloved Empire City gets to the second bar, the curious stranger inevitably asks that one question that makes all splendor vanish. It is a gut-wrenching question whose answer holds enough power to make you rise early to try to change the world or to keep you awake at night because you have seen what the world is really like. It is a gut-wrenching question that makes you want to take a long drag from a cigarette or down a martini before you answer, even if you don't smoke or drink: "What was it like on September 11th?" Now that question has been replaced by another grim one: "What was it like during the worst part of the pandemic?" "It" in this context is a loaded signifier, with complex nuances embedded in the stranger's inquiry. "It" can mean the city, my experience, the experiences of New Yorkers, and all of those things at once. However, I now realize that "it" also refers to a collective, primary need to understand how one endures an unthinkable, global tragedy, and how one protects one's self and family – ultimately, it becomes a question about survival.

While both questions remain painful, I no longer consider either to be insensitive or intrusive. They are, in fact, necessary. The City of New York is forever a microcosm of America that encapsulates all of our grit, gumption,

DOI: 10.4324/9781003400356-1

greed, and even generosity. Our glory and tragedy belong to everyone. New York is the place where "There is nothing that you can't do" (Shuckburgh et al., 2009) and where "If you can make it here, you can make it anywhere" (Sinatra et al., 1977).[1] At its core, New York is about survival. This book is about those New Yorkers, living in their concrete jungle, who plan to survive no matter what.

"Don't Panic," read the title of the 2020 March issue of *New York* magazine (Haskell, 2020). As the COVID-19 pandemic swept through the city, "panic" accurately summed up the collective feeling in New York. On a particularly gray day, someone had posted copies of this magazine cover, taped to lampposts throughout my Greenwich Village neighborhood. As I stood on line outside of Citarella, a neighborhood grocery store, I stared at that word, "panic," and tried not to. Scanning the line of masked New Yorkers, I reminded myself that New Yorkers were tough and that we just needed to hang on for a few more weeks. As it turned out, I probably should not have been so optimistic. During the pandemic, we, as a city, held steady for over 3 years. As of 2023, the city has had more than 3.25 million cases of COVID-19 (including the Delta, Omicron and BA.2 variants) and has suffered the loss of 45,123 New Yorkers (*New York Times*, n.d.).

New York's tenure as the first epicenter of the COVID-19 pandemic in the United States was a swift and brutal introduction to the virus's power to destroy the city by taking lives, upending the economy, and intensifying racial and class disparities. From mid-March until the end of June 2020 (the height of the pandemic), the virus had ravaged the city, with more than 215,000 confirmed cases, and over 23,000 deaths, representing 8% of confirmed cases in the United States, 18% of deaths domestically, and 5% globally (Partnership for New York City, 2020b). With nearly 1.6 million unemployment applications filed, the city's unemployment rate reached 19.8% (Partnership for New York City, 2020a). As New York's economy began to recover, lost tax revenue in the state and the city was anticipated to exceed $37 billion in the following two fiscal years (Partnership for New York City, 2021).

The COVID-19 pandemic has also exposed New York's staggering inequalities. As a global capital with a diverse population and a complex economy, the city's sharp divisions of class and race have been mirrored in the pandemic's impact. Beyond age, one's race and income were the most significant factors in determining one's chances for surviving the pandemic (Schwirtz & Rogers-Cook, 2020). In keeping with a pattern that occurred across the United States (Tai et al., 2021), New York City's racial and ethnic minority neighborhoods were disproportionately burdened by COVID-19 cases and deaths (Do & Frank, 2021). Fueled by factors such as employment in businesses that required face-to-face contact and inequalities in social and economic conditions, COVID-19 cases and deaths for majority Black, Latinx and other minority communities ranged between 24%

and 110% higher than those in majority White communities (Do & Frank, 2021). At the height of the pandemic, Blacks and Latinx residents were hospitalized and dying at twice the rate of Whites and Asians (Mays & Newman, 2020).

In the city's COVID-19 epicenter of Central Queens, the virus disproportionately affected working-class immigrants (Correal et al., 2020). Within these diverse immigrant communities, infection rates escalated among residents due to factors including suffering from preexisting chronic conditions, lacking health insurance, dealing with language barriers, living in crowded housing, working in high-exposure essential jobs, and enduring high rates of unemployment. Shielded by its wealth, Manhattan had the lowest death rates, as the rich left the city. At the start of the pandemic, the residential population of the borough's wealthiest neighborhoods like the Upper East Side, Soho, the West Village, and Brooklyn Heights decreased by 40% or more (Quealy, 2020). As Inez Barron, a city councilwoman whose Brooklyn district includes the ZIP code with the highest death rate in the city, observed, "We may all be in the same storm, but we're all not in the same boat" (Schwirtz & Rogers-Cook, 2020).

An analysis of the New York City Department of Health and Mental Hygiene (NYCDOH, 2021b) data on the COVID-19 death rate indicates that the Hispanic/Latino (32.34%) and the Black/African-American (30.68%) communities have suffered the highest death rates, at 63.02%, compared with the death rate of Whites (18.97%) and of Asians/Pacific-Islanders (18.01%). The uneven social and spatial distribution of confirmed COVID cases and deaths in New York has been driven mainly by social vulnerability, indicated by factors such as poverty, race, lack of health insurance, language impairment, and overcrowded living conditions (McPhearson et al., 2020).

These social vulnerabilities proved dangerous even prior to the COVID-19 outbreak. Based on the data obtained from the *2018 New York City Community Health Survey*, Arasteh (2021) found that Latinx immigrants were 46.5 times more likely to live in a neighborhood with high poverty, eight times more likely not to be undernourished in the previous 6 months and 1.4 times more likely to lack health insurance coverage, compared to US-born Whites. The unequal COVID-19 burden of New York's minority communities is also closely linked to employment (Do & Frank, 2021). According to the NYCDOH (2021a) data, three-quarters of New York's essential workers, including direct-service workers in grocery, pharmacy, transit, delivery, cleaning, healthcare, and social services, are people of color, and more than half were born outside of the United States. During the pandemic, Latinx and Black New Yorkers have been 1.3 to 2 times more likely than White New Yorkers to report financial hardships such as being unable to pay even for basic necessities, including rent or mortgage, gas, groceries, and phone service (NYCDOH, 2021b). Furthermore, NYCDOH reports that the inequities of experiences in this pandemic are consistent with past public health experiences and many chronic diseases.

COVID-19 also ravaged New York's economy. As a global city, New York is recognized as a financial and cultural nexus for the world. According to the Office of the New York State Comptroller (2020), New York's economy in 2019 was a juggernaut with the service economy, which includes finance and real estate, business services, tourism industries, and media, comprised nearly 70% of the city's 4.635 million jobs. At that time, New York was predicted to be the largest urban economy in the world by 2035 with the largest finance and business services sector (Holt, 2018). However, in 2020, among the 20 largest cities in the United States, New York lost the greatest share of jobs (11.8%) due to the pandemic, nearly three times the loss experienced at the national level (4.3%) (Parrott, 2021).

One of the most revealing pieces of data on the importance of New York's economic recovery (as well as fears about its fragility) was the creation of the "New York Recovery Index" in the financial website *Investopedia*, aired by television channel NY1. Calculated weekly and monthly, the "New York Recovery Index" was a composite score based on a combination of six sub-indices: COVID-19 Hospitalizations, Unemployment Claims, Home Sales, Rental Inventory, Subway Mobility, and Restaurant Reservations (Silver, July 2020a). The baseline score was 100 which reflected the health of the city's economy prior to the pandemic. The New York Recovery Index was first reported in July 2020, shortly after the worst months of the pandemic. Following the horrific consequences for both human life and on the city's economy, New York's score was 23. The August 2020 report (Silver, 2020b) emphasized the national significance of a strong New York economy:

> With an $86 billion annual budget – the largest of any city in the country – the loss of tax revenue from traditional sources of income will be felt for years to come. New York City's GDP is an impressive $1.5 trillion, so the city has an outsized influence on the country's overall economic health.

At the end of 2022, New York seemed poised for recovery with the city's final rating at 76 (Silver, 2022). However, the change from commuting to working remotely for so much of New York's workforce has threatened the revival of the city's economy. The demand for office space and the number of commuters to the city sharply declined, rather than rebounding to pre-pandemic levels, as many companies continued to allow remote work even after the danger had passed. In July 2021, 18.7% of all Manhattan office space was available for lease – more than double the pre-pandemic levels; it was, in fact, the highest rate on record (Haag, 2021). During this period, in an analysis of the 22 major office markets in the United States, New York was ranked last (22/22) based on the city's decline in commercial real estate leasing and investment, overall capital markets, retail, and economic rankings (Newmark, 2021). A qualifier explaining New York's ranking points to the difficulties of making predictions about the global capital's future economy:

> While [New York's] challenges are not insignificant, attention-grabbing headlines about the death of major cities are vastly overstated, as many of the metrics that placed New York at the bottom of the pack are temporary factors influenced by the pandemic.
>
> *(Newmark, 2021, p. 28)*

The qualifier is accurate. Although New York, one of America's great cities, is not dead, its economy is clearly changing. The drive behind this change can now be encapsulated in a single sentence: In 2023, New York City's vacant office space could fill 26.6 Empire State Buildings (Glaeser & Ratti, 2023).

In addition to the quantitative measures showing New York's staggering death toll and the colossal economic impact, to fully understand the pandemic's effect on New York, we must also examine the pandemic's effect on the everyday lives of New Yorkers – the lived experience (Lefebvre, 1991). The New York urban prepping community provides a special lens into the lived experience of New Yorkers devoted to preparing for crisis and can teach urban dwellers much about surviving a pandemic. Prepping refers to planning independently to survive disaster with scarce food and supplies, and in the absence of government aid (Mills, 2018). Prepping is an act of community resilience; its practices center on withstanding shocks and stresses by learning survival skills, adaptation, and thriving in harsh circumstances.[2] The philosophy of preparedness encompasses protecting one's family from disaster, homesteading, and sustainability. Preppers' belief in self-reliance, approaches to survival (sheltering in place or leaving the city), gathering resources (supplies and skills), and networking demonstrate capacities of community resilience (Faulkner et al., 2018).

Drawing on community resilience literature, this book offers a detailed qualitative analysis of the impact of the COVID-19 pandemic on New York City and on the philosophy and practices of the city's urban prepper subculture. With a special focus on the height of the pandemic in New York (from mid-March through June 2020), primary themes of the book include (1) examining New York's unique position as a global capital which made it the pandemic's first epicenter in the United States; (2) exploring the lived experience of enduring the pandemic by analyzing responses to the pandemic in the city as reflections of class division – in broad terms, the exodus of the wealthy, sheltering in place for the middle class, and the inability to leave high-risk neighborhoods for the poor – and by studying the sheltering-in-place practices as well as community resilience efforts by New York preppers; and (3) analyzing the importance of good government and an engaged citizenry in developing an agenda for the city's continued recovery and its future. These findings underscore the need for cities to develop disaster management approaches that expand traditional "command and control" models to make space for local knowledge and resources. At its core, this book is about understanding New York City's pandemic experience and how self-reliance evolves into community resilience outside of institutions.

This book is singular because it focuses on preppers trying to survive disaster rather than training for survival. In their pre-pandemic training for survival, most New York preppers learned both wilderness survival and sheltering-in-place skills. However, they believed that, in the next great disaster, they would have to abandon the city. Instead, the pandemic forced them to rely on their sheltering-in-place skills and adapt to a long-term crisis rather than an immediate one. Just like everyone else, New York preppers stepped into their new roles as telecommuters, teachers, caregivers, and counselors. Furthermore, their collective pandemic experience reinforced their philosophy of self-reliance. For urban preppers, the federal government's failure to enact a clear response to the pandemic reaffirmed their core belief that government could not be depended on in a time of crisis. These New Yorkers are not alone in their belief in the need for self-reliance. More than 11.4 million Americans report being prepared to survive independently for at least 31 days (Ellis, 2021).

This book builds on my ethnography of New York preppers (2017–2020) that drew from participant observations, interviews, and archival research. My book, *Bracing for the Apocalypse: An Ethnographic Study of New York's "Prepper" Subculture* (Bounds, 2020), explores the rise of the urban preppers' subculture in New York, shedding light on the distinctive approach of city dwellers in preparing for disaster. My book is the first ethnography about urban preppers. While research does exist on survivalist fringe groups that support specific political manifestos, my book is unique as it concerns mainstream urban preppers – those who seek to protect their families from the increasing risks of climate change, technological failure, epidemics or pandemics, and government or economic collapse. Drawing on symbolic interaction theory, my study analyzes the social structure of the city's only publicly known prepping group (New York City Preppers Network (NYCPN)) to discover how its practices reinforce a commitment to self-reliance. After conducting nearly three years of participant-observer research, my findings provide new insight on preppers. First, I have discovered that many New Yorkers have become interested in prepping based on their direct experience with disaster or disruption in the city. Second, New York preppers are a diverse group. They are billionaires. They are the working poor. They are often people of color. They are also often women. Their diverse identities shatter the media trope of a prepper as an isolated, rural, White male preoccupied with gun ownership. Stereotypical preppers worry about what the government has in store for them. Urban preppers, on the other hand, worry that the government has *nothing* in store for them (Suspicion confirmed!).

Literature on the growing phenomenon of prepping is only now emerging. Mills (2018) examines the influence of the media and politics on prepping. Through conducting interviews with American preppers and analyzing survey data, Mills's upcoming book analyzes prepping throughout the United States to understand the motivations behind preparedness. He argues that the increasing interest in prepping reflects an interaction between the United States' long-running valorization of self-reliant individualism and several aspects of contemporary social change in the early 21st century: surging fears of foreign and terrorist attacks after 9/11, growing distrust of federal emergency management, and the ascent of radical right-wing ideologies that have encouraged many Americans to interpret many political events (including the elections of Barack Obama and Joe Biden) as precipitating some kind of major social collapse. Drawing from in-depth interviews with preppers, Barker (2022) argues that prepper "awakening" narratives – the moment preppers "wake up" to the reality of crisis – spark an unusual form of agency. After recognizing their loss of security and increased vulnerability, individuals turn to self-reliance for protection rather than advocating for political or social change to re-establish their sense of safety. In studying the reinvention of bunkers and the renewed interest in hunkering down to escape the dangers of contemporary life, Garrett (2020) argues that prepping is a response to the instabilities of flawed political and social systems. According to Garrett (2020, p. 16), "Preppers do what they do whether it be stockpiling food or building a bunker [because] action provides solace." However, as the work of New York preppers during the pandemic will demonstrate, their activities are also practical tools of resilience.

It is clear that both Americans who identify as preppers and other Americans are now investing in emergency preparedness. Prepping is now a major force in American retail. One-third of American adults (about 74 million Americans) spent $11 billion in the last year on emergency preparedness (Laycock, 2023). The top five most commonly purchased items were food, water, toilet paper, medical supplies, and survival/emergency kits. Particularly trendy nowadays are pre-packaged emergency kits filled with basics such as flashlights, first aid supplies, and food and water rations. Emergency kit sales have been fueled by both the pandemic and the threat of natural disasters. Ready America, an emergency kit manufacturer, reports growth of 83% between 2017 and 2022, with Tropical Storm Hilary in California boosting the sales of its emergency backpack by 350% and emergency power station sales by 2,300% (Rothenberg, 2023). They are purchased mainly by people who are not interested in or uncertain about selecting their own items (non-preppers or new preppers, for example).

Preppers believe in carefully curating their own bug out bags and prepper closets. Beyond choosing their own tools and provisions, they are also committed to cultivating their knowledge of survival training and homesteading skills, and exploring wellness practices and alternative medicines. Therefore, the preparedness market is not relegated only to equipment like survival tools and ready-made emergency kits. Rather, the preparedness market is vast, encompassing other markets, ranging from wilderness survival schools and camping gear to athletic wear, bunkers, and essential oils. Lastly, to provide a different context for understanding consumer spending in the prepper market, it is worth noting a story of one hard-working and earnest entrepreneur who dedicated their life to starting a preparedness supply website just a few years before the pandemic. We have stayed in contact throughout my research. When I first spoke with him, I was impressed by his authenticity. For him, the world had become an increasingly risky place, and there was a need to be met. Since that first meeting, he has been a fully focused entrepreneur. By helping people better protect themselves during the pandemic, this entrepreneur has now been able to provide for his family and to pursue worthwhile projects. Due to his success, he also now owns a plane and more than one exotic sports car.

Weeks before the pandemic hit New York, Jason Charles, leader of the NYCPN explained, "Look, as preppers, we aren't freaked out about the pandemic. This is something that we have trained for. We already know how to shelter in place. We have our provisions. We know what to do." To those unfamiliar with prepping, his statement may seem bold; however, it reflects the philosophy of self-reliance inherent in the prepping culture. Based on the belief that the government will be unable to aid its citizens during a grave disaster, preppers support a philosophy of self-reliance that encompasses protecting one's families from disaster, engaging in homesteading and practicing sustainability. Echoing Emerson's (1841) sentiment, "Trust thyself. . . . Nothing is at last sacred but the integrity of your own mind." Preppers work hard to become more self-reliant by honing their survival knowledge and skill sets. Strengthening one's self-reliance involves mastering three areas: protecting one's family from disaster (sheltering in place or leaving the city), practicing homesteading, and engaging in sustainability. Throughout the pandemic, their efforts to improve their knowledge base, to network, and to gather resources (supplies and skills) demonstrated capacities of community resilience (Faulkner et al., 2018). Their disaster-preparedness training provided them with a plan for surviving the crisis. By practicing self-reliance, New York preppers step out of the traditional role of city dwellers in order to prevent themselves from being overtaken by the circumstances of disaster.

Staying in your home during a disaster is known as "sheltering in place." As described by the Department of Homeland Security (2019), "There may be situations, depending on your circumstances and the nature of the disaster, when it's simply best to stay where you are and avoid any uncertainty outside by 'sheltering in place.'" To store food and supplies, many New York preppers have dedicated spaces in their apartments that contain emergency supplies to help their families survive in dire circumstances. Such a storage area is referred to as a "prepper closet," which contains essentials such as medical supplies, protective equipment, nonperishable food, large containers of water, flashlights, and batteries. Prepper closets also contain special items for family members such as games or books for children as well as treats for adults (such as special snacks or alcohol). Typically, a prepper closet contains supplies for at least 1 month. At the start of the COVID-19 pandemic, New York preppers were already prepared to shelter in place with their prepper closets stocked with provisions required during a pandemic which included masks, gloves, protective clothing, and hand sanitizer. (They even know how to make hand sanitizer and how to filter water.)

For New York preppers, the philosophy of self-reliance is rooted in a sense of place – their experience of living in the city. According to Tuan (1975, p. 156), cities are "central to meaning." What meaning does New York have for these urban preppers in relation to planning for disaster? Urban prepping is about adapting to the changing nature of life as a city dweller. It is about the local, everyday choices, planning for the future, and thinking about community. As explained by one *New York Times* reader on the impact of COVID-19 on New York: "Being a New Yorker takes work." What is the work of community resilience? Norris et al. (2008) posit the following:

> To build collective resilience, communities must reduce risk and resource inequities, engage local people in mitigation, create organizational linkages, boost and protect social supports, and plan for not having a plan, which requires flexibility, decision-making skills, and trusted sources of information that function in the face of unknowns.
>
> *(p. 127)*

As COVID-19 tore through the city in late March 2020, Governor Andrew Cuomo sought to boost the morale of New Yorkers by reminding them of their steeliness. In one of his daily television press conferences, Cuomo (2020) told New Yorkers:

> We're going to get through it because we are New York and because we've dealt with a lot of things, and because we are smart. You have to be smart to make it in New York. And we are resourceful, and we are showing how resourceful we are. And because we are united, and when you are united, there is nothing you can't do. And because we are New York tough. We are tough. You have to be tough. This place makes you tough, but it makes you tough in a good way.

While Cuomo's words were intended to steady the nerves of an anxious public, his statement emphasized the fact that living in New York in the 21st century is, in fact, tough. Since the start of this century, New York has endured significant disasters (or threats of disasters) that make up the main categories of concern for urban preppers: terrorist attacks, technological failures, natural disasters, government or economic collapse, and pandemics (see Table 1.1). Manhattan has experienced five terrorist attacks in the 21st century: the World Trade Center attack (2001), the failed car bombing of Times Square (2010), the Chelsea bomb explosion (2016), the truck driven into people on West Side bike path (2017), and the Times Square-Port Authority subway bomb partial-detonation (2017). New York was battered by Hurricane Sandy (2012), the worst storm in the city's history. The Northeastern Blackout (2003) left New Yorkers without electricity for nearly 2 days, including thousands who were without mass transit. The Great Recession (2008) spun the city into an economic crisis. Also, as an international gateway, New York has always been in danger of the possible outbreak of pandemics or epidemics. While the city did not have significant outbreaks of Zika (2016) or Ebola (2014), New York endured an outbreak of the H1N1 influenza (the Swine Flu) in 2009. These direct experiences with disaster motivated many New Yorkers to learn prepping skills.

For New York, as the first epicenter of COVID-19, and for the United States, the devastating impact of COVID-19 across all areas of life (health, economic, and social) increased, due in large part to the federal government's failure to launch a comprehensive plan to battle COVID-19 (Slavitt, 2021). Serious policy mistakes can be traced throughout the chronology of the virus's spread, including President Donald Trump's decision to downplay early warnings about the virus, the lack of a national stockpile of protective equipment, the failure to coordinate a national supply chain for protective equipment and medical supplies, and the shifting policies on the wearing of face masks (Shear & McNeil, 2020). For New York preppers, the breakdown in governmental response at the federal level confirmed their belief in self-reliance. One prepper argued that the federal government's inability to manage the COVID crisis resulted in "a game of 'Whac-A-Mole' where problems related to the virus and confusion keep popping up."

As President Trump continued to deny the effects of the pandemic, a weary city turned its eyes toward Governor Andrew Cuomo of New York State. Under Cuomo's direction (and often at odds with Mayor Bill de Blasio), the New York State and New York City governments sought to address critical healthcare challenges (bed shortages, overwhelmed hospital staff, and a shortage of personal protective equipment for hospital workers) and guide to global capital through the process of sheltering in place. However, Cuomo's management style – namely, his need for complete control – often caused conflict with Mayor Bill de Blasio. As this book will

TABLE 1.1 New York City's Disasters and Disruptions

Terrorist attack	*Natural disaster*	*Pandemic/epidemic threat*	*Technological failure*	*Govt or economic instability*
2017 – Port Authority Terminal Bomb Attack 2017 – West Side Bike Path Vehicular Attack 2016 – Chelsea Bomb Attack 2010 – Time Square Bomb Attack 2001 – World Trade Center Attack	2017 – Winter Storm Stella 2017 – Winter Storm Niko 2016 – Flash Flood 2015 – Blizzard – Juno 2012 – Hurricane Sandy 2012 – Tornado, Waterspout 2011 – Hurricane Irene 2011 – Earthquake 2004 – Tropical Depression Ivan 2004 – Severe Storms and Flooding 2003 – Severe Storms, Tornadoes and Flooding 2002 – Earthquake	2020–2023 – COVID-19 2016 – Zika Virus Threat 2015 – Legionnaires Disease Outbreak 2015 – Measles Threat 2015 –Hepatitis A Threat 2014 – Ebola Virus Threat	2016 – East Harlem Metro North Train Fire 2016 – East Village Gas Explosion 2007 – Steam Pipe Explosion 2006 – Queens Blackout 2003 – Northeastern Blackout	2009 – The Great Recession 2008 – The Great Recession 2007 – The Great Recession

recount, these political battles – turf wars caused by the Governor's claim of sovereignty over the city – sometimes caused dangerous delays in protecting New Yorkers.

The pandemic has had a more significant impact on the city than the 9/11 terrorist attack, the Great Recession, or Hurricane Sandy (Partnership for New York City, 2020b). To tell this story, data for this project was collected through in-depth interviews, participation-observation, and online archival research. To develop an understanding of how New York preppers prepared for and lived during the pandemic, I conducted 40 interviews with New York City preppers, including members of two urban prepping groups, the NYCPN and Urban and Outdoor Survival (UOS), as well as independent preppers. Both the 486-member NYCPN and the 153-member UOS learn and practice preparedness strategies through lectures, workshops, and excursions. I attended online meetings of the NYCPN as an academic researcher. I also interviewed "independent preppers" (preppers not connected with any prepping group) across the five boroughs who maintained substantial provisions to hedge against disaster. While they may attend classes or events related to prepping, independent preppers do not train with a group. In fact, they do not plan to survive with or gain assistance from anyone beyond their close circle of family and close friends. Independent preppers have a wide range of incomes – from modest to extremely wealthy. I also talked with two high-net-worth (HNW) preppers about their pandemic experiences. As city prepper networks often have both residents and commuters as members, I spoke with preppers from New Jersey and Long Island, as well. To assess demand for prepping goods and services, I also interviewed owners of popular prepping gear websites.

Interview questions were designed to address the following broad categories: approaches to surviving the pandemic (such as sheltering in place or leaving the city), prepping skills and equipment that were most useful, unexpected challenges during the pandemic, the use of community networks for exchanging information and providing assistance, perceptions of life during the pandemic, and preparations or adjustments for continuing to endure the pandemic. These urban preppers' experiences offer valuable insight into understanding the broader experience of New Yorkers living in America, their first COVID-19 epicenter, and discovering possible community resilience strategies for city dwellers.

My archival research involved analyzing three categories of documents: (1) reports on the disasters in New York, including COVID-19's effect on poor and immigrant communities, (2) media coverage of New York preppers and prepping strategies, and (3) New York preppers' social media posts about prepping practice. The first category consists of policy documents and televised presentations by government officials and federal, state, and local agencies, reports published by nonprofit organizations such as community advocacy and public health organizations, press coverage of the COVID-19 pandemic's effect on poor and immigrant communities, and historical records of past epidemics in New York. Media coverage of New York preppers and prepping strategies during the pandemic include print, digital services, podcasts, and television. New York preppers' social media posts refer to public communication such as group Facebook pages, Instagram feeds, and Twitter messages.

My experience living through multiple crises as a New Yorker, which includes my sheltering-in-place experience during the COVID-19 pandemic for over 100 days, and enduring previous crises such as Hurricane Irene and Hurricane Sandy, as well as three terrorist attacks, has given me a unique perspective as a researcher. The primary aim of this study has been to examine how urban preppers have utilized their prepping skills and knowledge to survive the pandemic and how they plan to hone their approaches to improve their respective quality of life as the pandemic continues. Yet, my subject position as a New Yorker experiencing the pressures caused by the pandemic forced me to contend with the challenges of conducting fieldwork and even maintaining everyday life in dangerous circumstances that threatened to replace order and control with chaos and vulnerability (Nilan, 2002). As I supported my students through tremendous losses and as I witnessed the warp-speed demise of my neighborhood, maintaining the ethnographer's simultaneous role of being detached yet engaged (Willson, 1995, p. 255) sometimes felt less like a measured approach and more like a tightrope walk. In this regard, my research also draws on autoethnography. By discussing some of my significant personal experiences of sheltering-in-place in a detailed and deliberate way, I hope to accomplish the work of autoethnography by offering insight into "the emotional and relational aspects of culture and social life as well as providing an approach for grappling with the everyday and emergent aspects of the lived experience" (Holman Jones & Adams, 2023; p. 987) during lockdown in Manhattan.

In my first podcast interview about preppers and the pandemic, my voice cracked when discussing COVID's devastation of certain sections of Queens. I had been invited to discuss my research but I was overwhelmed with fear and sadness for my friends and students who resided in these areas. After that interview, I came to understand the importance of "becoming-with" in research, embracing the personal and valuing our connections and how we relate to one another Throughout this project, the lyrics of Coldplay's "The Scientist" have come to mind more than once: "I was just guessing at numbers and figures/Pulling the puzzles apart/Questions of science, science and progress/Do not speak as loud as my heart" (Coldplay, 2002). As a city and as a nation, we have experienced great tragedy. To strengthen our resiliency, our story of survival must be told – a story of adapting, rebuilding, and reimagining. To get at the hope, we also have to bear witness.

My research finds that prepping is not merely evidence of the American belief in the power of the individual but an expression of urban citizenship that is grounded in a loss of faith in government support and a turn toward local bonds that foster resiliency. As this book will discuss, for urban preppers, their identities as New Yorkers and attachment to their city were sources of strength and resilience in coping with the threat of COVID-19. During the pandemic, urban preppers bolstered community resilience by relying on prepping strategies to protect themselves and shelter in place more effectively, sharing their knowledge and resources with their neighbors. Their philosophy of self-reliance has helped them to survive the pandemic and brace for future surges. However, as noted by the Partnership for New York City (2020a), "The pandemic unleashed political, racial and economic tensions that can either leave in chaos the nation's largest and most important urban center, or . . . provide the impetus for working together for recovery and positive change." Now, survival is dependent on the resilience of the city.

The resilience of New York depends on good government initiatives, the support of the business and nonprofit sectors, civic leaders, and an engaged citizenry. In "prepper" terminology, a "bug out" plan to escape the impact of this crisis is necessary. As de Blasio ended his final term as mayor, his contribution to directing a way forward for the city never materialized. In 2021, Eric Adams, former New York State Senator and former New York Police Department captain, was elected as mayor, running on safety and crime reduction platforms. A crucial missing item from the new mayor's agenda was a clear plan for recovery that involves working toward decreasing social vulnerabilities – the social, cultural, and economic factors that shape a group's ability to respond to and recover from disaster (Masterson et al., 2014). In 2023, that plan is still missing. Furthermore, at the state level, Governor Cuomo's resignation due to sexual harassment allegations in 2021 was shocking. His replacement, Lt. Governor Kathy Hochul, has seemed to be more of a consensus-builder and less aggressive in working with colleagues, which is a clear asset, but she has inherited incredible challenges. However, an end to the Cuomo era, and to the Cuomo–de Blasio conflict, has somewhat strengthened the city's position in working with New York state. As noted by State Senator Liz Krueger, a Democrat from Manhattan, "His [Cuomo's] existence and the way he liked to function was to establish extreme levels of stress and tension. Almost anyone else would not be the same zeitgeist for the city" (Ferre-Sadurni, 2021).

During the height of the pandemic, an urban prepper with a keen sense of humor recently posted a meme on social media that read: "Someone asked if I had plans for the fall." (Depending on one's interpretation, the word "fall" could be defined either as "Autumn" or "the collapse of civilization"). The joke also made me think about the "in-betweenness" of this book. Writing a book about the lived experience of New Yorkers amid the COVID-19 crisis is a fraught process. New York is always changing. Life is always changing. However, as a symbol of the city's energy and regeneration, New York preppers continue to develop new strategies for survival based on their experiences enduring COVID-19 to protect their families and aid their communities.

Following Chapter 1's introductory framework for examining the pandemic's impact on the philosophy and practices of New York's urban prepper subculture, Chapter 2, "History of Contagions and Chaos in the City," establishes a context for understanding New York's significance as a global city and COVID-19's place in New York's history of disaster. This chapter traces how the city's lack of stability was due not only to the intensity of the pandemic but also to rising tensions between different levels of government (federal, state, and city). At the core of this narrative is the diminished belief in government's ability or interest in aiding its citizens. Central to the COVID-19 discussion is the profound impact of the federal government's failure to develop a clear and comprehensive national plan to protect its citizens as well as the struggle for control of the city between Governor Andrew Cuomo and Mayor Bill de Blasio. The chapter analyzes the spread of COVID-19 throughout the city, identifying local governmental efforts to slow the spread, the health crisis as patient numbers skyrocketed, and the devastating impact on poor communities of color (the epicenter within the epicenter). The chapter also discusses how, in the months preceding COVID-19's arrival in the city, New York preppers set about to protect their families against the virus and to prepare to shelter in place.

Chapter 3, "Escape from New York: When the Rich Left the City," analyzes the narratives surrounding the abandonment of the city by wealthy residents at the start of the pandemic. In the event of a grave disaster, New York's wealthy preppers had already planned to escape the city for their strategic relocation destinations (posh retreats in exotic locales). However, amplifying the sharp class division within cities, the majority of New York's wealthy also fled the city. Exploring the real and feared consequences offers insight into how this exodus of over 400,000 rich residents, mainly from Manhattan, represents the ever-increasing polarization between classes in the city. Perspectives on this issue from New Yorkers who remained in the city during the pandemic are shared to study the cultural significance of wealthy residents' departures (and delayed returns) to the city such as fears of white flight and an impending financial crisis. The next section discusses the significant pressure that their relocation had on their new homes as New York's wealthy shifted from temporary visitors to permanent residents, creating soaring housing costs, congestion, demands on healthcare and food supplies, and overwhelming school systems. The chapter closes by arguing that the departure from the city by the extremely wealthy and their seamless relocation to safe havens reflects the inequality of "the velvet rope economy" that has allowed America's rich to glide past the dangers and inconveniences endured by ordinary Americans (Schwartz, 2020).

Chapters 4 and 5 of this book explore NYC preppers' experiences of sheltering in place in the city – from planning for the pandemic to enduring the struggles of living through an extended period of confinement. Chapter 4 explores prepping as a lifestyle that requires a commitment to learning and readiness. It also describes the strategies of sheltering in place, such as the mastery of homesteading and first aid skills. It also explores the significance of the prepper closet as a critical tool for survival. Chapter 5 discusses the challenges and success of New York preppers' sheltering-in-place experiences. First, the chapter examines the response of preppers to the management of the pandemic by government. Next, it looks at the importance of preparedness strategies during the pandemic, such as the significance of the prepper closet to households and the value of networks to secure information and resources. Lastly, the chapter examines the challenges experienced by preppers.

In the spirit of trying to figure out "how" and "why" being part of a community is so beneficial, Chapter 6 explores prepping in New York City as an act of community resilience that seeks to strengthen preparedness and social networks as well addressing the inequitable distribution of resources during disaster. Drawing from Hall and Lamont, community resilience refers to a social group's ability "to sustain its well-being in the face of challenges" (Hall & Lamont, 2012, p. 232). Drivers of resilience are the experiences that group members hold in common as well as the organizational frameworks that form them. How does participation in a prepping group foster resiliency? By analyzing the rationale behind why New Yorker preppers prepare for disasters, we can see how community members actually take on the task of learning resiliency. Their belief in self-reliance, approaches to survival (sheltering in place or leaving the city), gathering resources (supplies and skills), and networking are important factors that help NYCPN members mobilize for action. The NYCPN is not posited as a model for forming community resiliency groups. Instead, my purpose is to explore the activities of this group for what it is – an authentic local response to survival in a city at increased risk.

To provide insight for developing an agenda for continued recovery and future responses to disaster, Chapter 7 draws from the philosophy of prepping to offer an alternative perspective for planning New York's future. The pandemic has demonstrated that practicing emergency preparedness was useful and that relying only on aid from the government during a crisis might be risky. As Ryan notes, resilience is best derived from both "top-down" approaches as well as "bottom-up" strategies and ordinary tactics (2015). Therefore, this chapter explores a list of prepper adages to consider in planning for New York's future. Urban preppers can teach us much about the benefits of self-reliance – networking and community-building in a period of crisis. Urban resiliency demands the foundation of both a dedicated community and a strong city government. Their practices are also potent reminders of the kind of power that an engaged citizenry can hold. Yet, their philosophy also underscores the distrust in government that is now commonplace among Americans.

Chapter 8 discusses NYC prepping practices first as possible local resiliency strategies, focusing on preparedness, adaptation, and community. This chapter also outlines the core components needed for strengthening the city's resiliency, purpose, evolution, and community-building. The book's close argues that good government and an engaged citizenry are vital to New York's future.

In a *New York Times* op-ed piece, Jerry Seinfeld identifies another critical element inherent in the city that will ensure its survival: its energy. Responding to those who argue that New York is now "dead," Seinfeld argues that the energy found in New York is what drives its resilience and its future. He refers to the energy found in cities; the spark ignites when city dwellers congregate. Seinfeld writes, "Energy, attitude and personality cannot be 're-moted' through even the best optic lines" and that this special quality is what continues to draw people to New York (2020, para.12). He is right. It is that city verve that Jane Jacobs wrote about so long ago:

> Dull, inert cities, it is true, do contain the seeds of their own destruction and little else. But lively, diverse, intense cities contain the seeds of their own regeneration, with energy enough to carry over for problems and needs outside themselves.
>
> *(1961, p. 448)*

In 2024, we are all still betting on Jacobs.

Notes

1 Liza Minelli actually first released "New York, New York" in 1977. Frank Sinatra released a cover of the song in 1979.
2 For a detailed analysis of community resilience definitions and measurements, see Wright (2022).

References

Arasteh, K. (2021). Hypertension, diabetes and poverty among Latinx immigrants in New York City: Implications for COVID-19. *International Journal of Migration, Health and Social Care*, 17(2), 208–241. https://doi.org/10.1108/IJMHSC-09-2020-0088

Barker, K. (2022). Awakening from the sleep-walking society: Crisis, detachment and the real in prepper awakening narratives. *Sage Journals*. https://doi.org/10.1177/02637758221123814

Bounds, A. M. (2020). *Bracing for the apocalypse: An ethnographic study of New York's "prepper" subculture*. Routledge.

Coldplay. (2002). *The scientist* [Song]. On a rush of blood to the head. Parlophone (UK). Capitol (US).

Correal, A., Jacobs, A., & Jones, R. C. (2020, April 9). "A tragedy is unfolding": Inside New York's virus epicenter. *The New York Times*. www.nytimes.com/2020/04/09/nyregion/coronavirus-queens-corona-jackson-heights-elmhurst.html

Cuomo, A. (2020, March 24). Video, audio, photos & rush transcript: Governor Cuomo: In New York, "Love wins and it will win again through this virus". *Governor of New York*. www.governor.ny.gov/news/video-audio-photos-rush-transcript-governor-cuomo-new-york-love-wins-and-it-will-win-again

Department of Homeland Security (DHS). (2019). *Planning considerations: Evacuation and shelter-in place guidance for state, local, tribal, and territorial partners*. www.fema.gov/sites/default/files/2020-07/planning-considerations-evacuation-and-shelter-in-place.pdf

Do, D. P., & Frank, R. (2021). Unequal burdens: Assessing the determinants of elevated COVID-19 case and death rates in New York City's racial/ethnic minority neighbourhoods. *Journal of Epidemiology and Community Health*, *75*(4), 321–326. https://doi.org/10.1136/jech-2020-215280

Ellis, C. M. (2021). *Are you ready for it? Examining security in contemporary disaster preparedness, from normal to Noachian* [Unpublished doctoral dissertation, Cornell University].

Emerson, R. W. (2001). Self-reliance (1841). In *Nature and selected essays*. Penguin Classics.

Faulkner, L., Brown, K., & Quinn, T. (2018). Analyzing community resilience as an emergent property of dynamic social-ecological systems. *Ecology and Society*, *23*(1). https://doi.org/10.5751/ES-09784-23012

Ferré-Sadurní, L. (2021, August 11). Hochul vows a change in tone as the Cuomo era nears an end in Albany. *The New York Times*. www.nytimes.com/2021/07/01/nyregion/manhattan-vacant-office-space-real-estate.html

Garrett, B. (2020). *Bunker: Building for the end times*. Scribner.

Glaeser, E., & Ratti, C. (2023, May 10). 26 Empire state buildings could fit into New York's empty office space. That's a sign. *The New York Times*. https://www.nytimes.com/interactive/2023/05/10/opinion/nyc-office-vacancy-playground-city.html

Haag, M. (2021, July 1). Office vacancies soar in New York, a dire sign for the city's recovery. *The New York Times*. www.nytimes.com/2021/07/01/nyregion/manhattan-vacant-office-space-real-estate.html

Haskell, D. (2020, March 16–29). Don't panic. *New York Magazine*. https://nymag.com/tags/don%27t-panic/

Holman Jones, S. H., & Adams, T. E. (2023). Autoethnography as being with. In N. K. Denzin & Y. S. Lincoln (Eds.), *The SAGE handbook of qualitative research* (6th ed.). Sage.

Holt, R. (2018). Global cities. Which cities will be leading the global economy in 2035? *thedialogue.org*. https://globaltrends.thedialogue.org/publication/which-cities-will-be-leading-the-global-economy-in-2035/

Jacobs, J. (1961). *The death and life of Great American cities*. Vintage Books.

Laycock, R. (2023, April 11). Doomsday preppers: How many are preparing for disaster? *Finder*. www.finder.com/doomsday-prepper-statistics

Lefebvre, H. (1991). *The production of space*. Wiley-Blackwell.

Masterson, J. H., Peacock, W. G., Van Zandt, S. S., Grover, H., Schwarz, L. F., & Cooper, J. T. Jr. (2014). *Planning for community resilience: A handbook for reducing vulnerability to disasters*. Island Press/Center for Resource Economics.

Mays, J. C., & Newman, A. (2020, April 8). Virus is twice as deadly for black and Latino people than whites in N.Y.C. *The New York Times*. www.nytimes.com/2020/04/08/nyregion/coronavirus-race-deaths.html

McPhearson, T., Grabowski, Z., Herreros-Cantis, P., Mustafa, A., Ortiz, L., Kennedy, C., Tomateo, C., Lopez, B., Olivotto, V., & Vantu, A. (2020). Pandemic injustice: Spatial and social distributions of COVID-19 in the US epicenter. *Journal of Extreme Events*, 7(4), 2150007. https://doi.org/10.1142/s234573762150007x

Mills, M. F. (2018). Preparing for the unknown . . . unknowns: "Doomsday" prepping and disaster risk anxiety in the United States. *Journal of Risk Research*, 1–13.

Newmark. (2021, June). The Newmark Opportunity Index: Identifying commercial real estate opportunities and challenges in major U.S. markets. *Newmark*. www.nmrk.com/storage-nmrk/uploads/fields/1-column-with-sidebar-links/Newmark_Opportunity_Index_June2021_2021_FINAL.pdf

New York City Department of Health and Mental Hygiene. (2021a, June 7). *COVID-19: Data NYC department of health and mental hygiene*. https://www1.nyc.gov/site/doh/covid/covid-19-data-totals.page

New York City Department of Health and Mental Hygiene. (2021b, June 7). *Inequities in experience of the COVID-19 pandemic, New York City*. https://www1.nyc.gov/assets/doh/downloads/pdf/epi/databrief123.pdf

New York Times. (n.d.). Tracking coronavirus in New York: Latest map and case count. *The New York Times*. www.nytimes.com/interactive/2021/us/new-york-covid-cases.html

Nilan, P. (2002). Dangerous fieldwork re-examined: The question of researcher subject position. *Qualitative Research*, *2*(3), 363–386.

Norris, F. H., Stevens, S. P., Pfefferbaum, B., Wyche, K. F., & Pfefferbaum, R. L. (2008). Community resilience as a metaphor, theory, set of capacities, and strategy for disaster readiness. *American Journal of Community Psychology*, *41*(1), 127–150.

Office of the New York State Comptroller. (2020). *Economic and demographic trends*. www.osc.ny.gov/reports/finance/2020-fcr/economic-and-demographic-trends

Parrott, J. A. (2021, May). NYC job losses proportionately greatest among largest U.S. cities. (CNYCA Econ Report). *Center for New York City Affairs at the New School*. www.centernyc.org/reports-briefs/2021/4/9/nyc-job-losses-proportionately-greatest-among-largest-us-cities

Partnership for New York City. (2020a). *A call for action and collaboration*. https://pfnyc.org/research/a-call-for-action-and-collaboration/

Partnership for New York City. (2020b, June). New York City COVID-19 economic impact update – Partnership for New York City. *Partnership for New York City*. https://pfnyc.org/research/new-york-city-covid-19-economic-impact-update/

Partnership for New York City/Department of Labor. (2021). *Signs of progress: NYC's economic recovery – Partnership for New York City*. https://pfnyc.org/research/signs-of-progress

Quealy, K. (2020, May 15). The richest neighborhoods emptied out most as coronavirus hit New York City. *The New York Times*. www.nytimes.com/interactive/2020/05/15/upshot/who-left-new-york-coronavirus.html

Rothenberg, E. (2023, August 26). Personal emergency kits are a growing market in an uncertain world. *CNN Business*. www.cnn.com/2023/08/26/business/emergency-disaster-kit-sales-climate/index.html

Schwartz, N. (2020). *The velvet rope economy: How inequality became big business*. Doubleday.

Schwirtz, M., & Rogers-Cook, L. (2020, June 22). These N.Y.C. neighborhoods have the highest rates of virus deaths. *The New York Times*. www.nytimes.com/2020/05/18/nyregion/coronavirus-deaths-nyc.html

Seinfeld, J. (2020, August 24). Opinion. *The New York Times*. www.nytimes.com/2020/08/24/opinion/jerry-seinfeld-new-york-coronavirus.html

Shear, M. D., & McNeil, D. G., Jr. (2020, April 14). Criticized for pandemic response, Trump tries shifting blame to the WHO. *The New York Times*. www.nytimes.com/2020/04/14/us/politics/coronavirus-trump-who-funding.html

Shuckburgh, A., Hunte, A., Keys, A., Keyes, B., Sewell-Ulepic, J., Carter, S., & Robinson, S. (2009). Empire state of mind [Recorded by Jay-Z & A. Keys] *On the Blueprint 3* [MP3]. Roc Nation.

Silver, C. (2020a, July 28). Tracking NYC's economic recovery from the coronavirus pandemic. *Investopedia*. Retrieved June 7, 2022, from www.investopedia.com/new-york-city-nyc-economic-recovery-index-5072042

Silver, C. (2020b, August 4). The New York City recovery index: Week of July 27. *Investopedia*. www.investopedia.com/nyc-recovery-index-archive-7-27-5073257

Silver, C. (2022, March 16). The New York City recovery index: March 7. *Investopedia*. www.investopedia.com/the-new-york-city-recovery-index-march-7-5222515

Sinatra, F., Kander, J., & Ebb, F. (1977). Theme from New York, New York. *Vocal Popular Sheet Music Collection*. Score 3274. https://digitalcommons.library.umaine.edu/mmb-vp-copyright/3274

Slavitt, A. (2021). *Preventable: The inside story of how leadership failures, politics, and selfishness doomed the U.S. coronavirus response*. St. Martin's Press.

Tai, D. B. G., Sia, I. G., Doubeni, C. A., & Wieland, M. L. (2022). Disproportionate impact of COVID-19 on racial and ethnic minority groups in the United States: A 2021 update. *Journal of Racial and Ethnic Health Disparities*, *9*(6), 2334–2339.

Tuan, Y. (1975). Place: An experiential perspective. *The Geographical Review*, *65*(2), 151–165. https://doi.org/10.2307/213970

Willson, M. (1995). Afterword perspective and difference: Sexualization, the field, and the ethnographer. In D. Kulick & M. Willson (Eds.), *Taboo: Sex, identity, and erotic subjectivity in anthropological fieldwork*. Routledge.

2

HISTORY OF CONTAGIONS AND CHAOS IN THE CITY

In September 2018, the Museum of the City of New York opened its "Germ City: Microbes and the Metropolis" exhibition, marking the centenary of the 1918 flu epidemic which killed 50 million people. Supported by The New York Academy of Medicine and Wellcome Foundation, the exhibition was the inaugural event of "Contagious Cities" – an international initiative designed to promote dialogue about the global challenges of epidemic preparedness and the role of cities in causing and combating infectious diseases (Moores, 2018).[1] During a press event for the exhibition's opening, Sarah M. Henry, Deputy Director and Chief Curator at the Museum of the City of New York, observed that "New York has always been a crossroads of people, goods and ideas, and also of germs" (Druckman & Young, 2021). Through a collection of visual artifacts juxtaposed against contemporary art, "Germ City" traced the complex history of New York's battle against infectious diseases. Medical equipment such as a gigantic Iron Lung, the size of a small submarine, reminded visitors of the tremendous difficulties of treating respiratory diseases in earlier eras. Simultaneously, the complexities and injustices related to treating disease were revealed by art works such as Ekene Ijeoma's "Pan-African AIDS," a series of sculptures (stacked plexiglass plates representing Africa and the United States) that explored "the hypervisibility of the HIV/AIDS epidemic in Africa and the hidden one in Black America" (Ijeoma, 2018, Studio). In the future, what social artifacts will be used to represent what life was like in New York during the COVID-19 pandemic? Perhaps photos of a desolate Times Square or of the diverse range of street art created during lockdown. Maybe video archives of the many livestream events presented by NYC's artists, dancers, and musicians during lockdown. Such an exhibition may even include original works by Governor Cuomo,

DOI: 10.4324/9781003400356-2

which included a television show, a tapestry of masks, a Styrofoam mountain, and a poster.[2]

With its mission to "reveal how our understanding of disease has changed us physically, socially, and culturally, and the surprising interplay between people and pathogens in an urban context" (Museum of the City of New York, 2018, Germ City), "Germ City" was a strangely accurate foreshadowing of the use of art as a rhetorical device to convey COVID-19's effect on New York at the height of the pandemic. Governor Andrew Cuomo (2011–2021) actually relied on two art forms to share information with New Yorkers (and the world) about the devastating effects of COVID during the first 100 days of the pandemic: a daily television show and a poster map. Drawing on the power of electronic media (television and the Internet) to attract viewers, Governor Cuomo gave daily televised press briefings that offered details about the number of positive diagnoses, the number of deaths, protection guidelines, and government measures undertaken to combat the virus. Harkening back to the political campaign posters of the 19th century, utilized before the advent of computer technology, Governor Cuomo commissioned "New York Tough," a curious poster map designed to reflect New York State's epic odyssey in overcoming COVID-19. While both artworks sparked controversy and endured a measure of disdain, Cuomo was awarded an Emmy for his televised press briefings, and his poster map was quite popular (Rosen, 2020). Despite their political leanings, these "artworks" did reveal how COVID was changing the city, physically, socially, and culturally. As a global capital, New York's stability would be defined by its success in stopping the spread of COVID-19 and in maintaining its tremendous economy. This chapter traces how the city's stability was rocked not only by the intensity of the pandemic but also by rising tensions between the federal, state, and city levels of government. At the core of this narrative is the diminished belief of preppers in government's ability or interest in aiding its citizens. In this context, New York preppers set about to protect their families against the virus and to prepare to shelter in place.

In early February 2020, New York was faced with the possible docking of a Royal Caribbean cruise ship with four passengers, all Chinese nationals, who showed symptoms of COVID-19 (Calfas, 2020). As Governor Cuomo (2020a, pp. 5–6) recalled:

> This was the first case that would come knocking on New York's door. In the end, the ship docked in Bayonne, New Jersey, and the four passengers who were transferred to a hospital for further evaluation tested negative, but the situation gave me the first true sense that we were on a journey to a place that we had never been before.

However, New York had already taken similar journeys to the edge of doom. In this 21st-century pandemic, we are not very different from our ancestors in that, at the beginning, we knew little about COVID-19, its mode of transmission, the human body's potential responses, and effective treatment options (Gordon, 2020). Consider the Yellow Fever Epidemic in New York. In 1793, Yellow Fever raged through Philadelphia, killing thousands. To prevent it from spreading to New York, ships from Philadelphia were quarantined. However, the brief quarantine only seemed to have postponed Yellow Fever's arrival, and from 1795 to 1804, Yellow Fever raged through the city (Weissman Center, 2010). The virus was transmitted by mosquitoes, a fact unknown at the time, and the hot, humid New York summer caused the rates of infection to spike. The rich fled the city, while many of those who remained suffered its horrendous symptoms ranging from yellowing of eyes and skin to delirium and seizures. As Winegard (2020, p. 3) notes, "Mosquitoes and other diseases that have accompanied traders, travelers, soldiers, and settlers around the world have been far more lethal than any man-made weapons or inventions."

One hundred and twenty-five years later, the 1918 Influenza pandemic caused 50 million deaths worldwide. At the height of this pandemic, New York City lost 31,589 people among its 5.5 million residents.[3] To place COVID-19 in a historical context of pandemics in New York City, the mortality associated with COVID-19 during the early phase of the New York City outbreak was comparable to the peak mortality observed during the 1918 Influenza pandemic (Faust et al., 2020). As an international gateway, New York's popularity has soared, along with its risk for spreading infectious diseases. In the decade preceding the pandemic, the Port Authority's airport system sets a record for its longest run of consecutive years of growth (an annual average of 3.3%) (Port Authority NY-NJ, 2020). In 2019, a record-breaking 140.5 million airline passengers, including 51 million international visitors, traveled through the region's airports (Port Authority NY-NJ, 2020). Given this tremendous number of passengers, New York's airport system was also a potential incubator and fast spreader of infectious diseases. For example, in 2016, New Yorkers faced the threat of the Zika virus, which causes severe birth defects in newborns whose mothers were infected while pregnant. The city had 987 cases of Zika with all cases linked to travel to a Zika-affected area (New York City Department of Health, 2019). In 2014, New York was also threatened by the Ebola virus at the height of the epidemic in West Africa. A New York doctor who treated patients with Ebola in Guinea contracted the virus upon his return to the city (Santora, 2014). After being isolated and treated for 19 days, the doctor recovered. The city also experienced an outbreak of the H1N1 influenza (Swine Flu) epidemic in 2009. To prevent the rapid spread of the influenza virus within the New York's public school system, 15 schools were closed throughout Queens and Brooklyn (Hartocollis, May 2009). H1N1 caused the death of 12 New Yorkers, including a Queens middle school principal, and an estimated 550,000 became sick (Hartocollis, June 2009).

New York's position as an international gateway was a contributing factor in the arrival of COVID-19 to the city. On March 1, Governor Cuomo had confirmed New York State's first case of COVID-19: a female healthcare worker who lived in Manhattan had contracted the virus while traveling in Iran (Goldstein, 2020). Less than 2 weeks later, New Rochelle, a suburb of the city, became a containment zone after an outbreak occurred at a religious event (Nir & Mckinley, 2020). Subsequent genome research revealed that the virus had actually arrived in New York by late January and most cases came from Europe (Zimmer, 2020). At the end of January 2020, President Trump had barred foreign nationals from entering the country if they had visited China within the previous 2 weeks. Visitors from most European countries were banned in mid-March. However, by the time the travel bans were implemented, COVID-19 had already landed in New York.

With the news of the first case, New York moved to the forefront in battling the pandemic. The New York State legislature granted Governor Cuomo emergency powers to lead the battle against the virus, which included issuing executive orders to close businesses and public schools. Governor Cuomo also began to hold daily televised press briefings to inform the public about the spread of the virus and the government's efforts to combat it. In a time of public fear and confusion regarding the federal government's lack of leadership in responding to the pandemic, his daily press briefings provided transparency and critical real-time updates, encouraged adherence to COVID-19 policies, and boosted morale. Each daily briefing followed the same format – a traditional PowerPoint presentation (with graphics often created by the Governor), a brief lecture, and personal reflections. Cuomo (2020a) viewed his daily briefings as an important policy tool for presenting data to the public in a way that was accessible but informational, and as a way to re-establish connection and trust between the public and government. His daily briefings were so central to America's conversation about COVID-19 that he was awarded an Emmy. As the president and CEO of the Academy of Television Arts and Sciences, Bruce Paisner, explained in a statement announcing the decision to award Governor Cuomo an Emmy:

> The Governor's 111 daily briefings worked so well because he effectively created television shows, with characters, plot lines, and stories of success and failure. People around the world tuned in to find out what was going on, and New York tough became a symbol of the determination to fight back.
>
> *(Dwyer, 2020, para. 4)*

Each episode worked to create a narrative that revealed the challenges of trying to manage the crisis in a context of conflict at all levels of government. Like many New Yorkers, I often received a phone call from a friend or colleague after each day's briefing to talk over his presentation. While mulling over the governor's analysis, we also shared our own news, which often centered around loss – the loss of lives, the loss of employment, and the loss of and longing for the energy and possibilities of pre-COVID New York. There may also have been a few conversations about fearing the loss of sanity.

Throughout the first brutal months of the pandemic, Cuomo's briefings also served as an ongoing discussion with President Trump. Depending on the briefings' content, Trump would subsequently rebuke or repeat analysis provided by Cuomo. COVID-19's catastrophic effect on the United States increased due to the federal government's failure to develop and execute a clear and coordinated plan for reducing the spread of virus across the country (Leonnig & Rucker, 2021). Well before the outbreak in 2018, the Trump Administration committed its first error when it eliminated the White House Pandemic Response Team. The nation's Strategic National Stockpile (SNS) was also neither strategic nor a stockpile. Established by Congress under the Bush Administration, the SNS was a repository of medical supplies, drugs, and vaccines to aid state and local governments during emergencies. Managed by the Department of Health and Human Services in coordination with the Department of Homeland Security, the SNS's success has been marred by complacency and a lack of political support since its creation. Slavitt (2021) reveals the impact of the federal government's failure to continue funding the SNS: To combat the Swine Flu epidemic in 2009, the SNS distributed 85 million N95 masks. In 2011, the Obama administration's request for funding to replenish the stockpile was denied by a Republican House that later reduced the stockpile's funding by 10%. Furthermore, the Obama administration's request for additional funding for the stockpile during the Zika and Ebola threats were reduced by half. Finally, the strategic plan for responding to a national emergency was not renewed during the Trump administration. At the beginning of the pandemic, the SNS's low inventory consisted of deteriorating masks or masks with expired usage dates and contained only about 12 million of the 3.5 billion N95 masks that were estimated to be needed for battling the pandemic (Slavitt, 2021). Ventilators and other protective personal equipment (PPE) were also in extremely short supply. The failure to invest in the replenishment of the SNS immediately eliminated the possibility of a swift federal response to the pandemic (Sanger et al., 2020). As Gordon (2020, p. 11) notes, "Pandemics are great for movies but not great for politics. When 'not in my lifetime' is a widely held belief, and political lives are measured in months not decades, politicians are disinclined to invest in a once-in-a century cataclysm."

New York's lack of access to a national stockpile resulted in a mad scramble to obtain additional medical supplies and personal protective equipment from the federal government and a heated conflict with President Trump. Rather than addressing the shortage of supplies in the national stockpile or aiding states in securing supplies from other resources, President Trump downplayed the virus and debated the need for requested items. These deflection tactics blocked efforts to aid those who had contracted the virus and to slow its spread. For example, in early March, Governor Cuomo requested 40,000 ventilators from the federal government based on an analysis by researchers from McKinsey & Co. and Cornell Medical School. President Trump's initial response was to push back by publicly doubting the need for the requested number of ventilators rather than supporting coordination between the two levels of government to address the shortage (Abutaleb & Paletta, 2021). As fears about the lack of ventilators began to transition into a public relations nightmare, the federal government supplied 700 ventilators initially, and then later, 4,000 ventilators in response to the state's immediate needs (Abutaleb & Paletta, 2021). However, there was also a lack of transparency about the size of and access to the New York State Emergency Stockpile. Regarding ventilators, President Trump fueled the suspicion on social media that New York was hoarding rather than using its stockpile, with messages like "New York had thousands of unused ventilators that needed to be distributed 'now!'" (Brown, 2020). Governor Cuomo argued that ventilators from the state's stockpile were being distributed based on immediate need (Lewis, 2020). Yet, during this same time period (late March 2020), the New York-Presbyterian Hospital began "ventilator sharing," treating two patients rather than one on a ventilator to help alleviate the shortage (Rosenthal et al., 2020).

Beyond the absence of a national stockpile, other critical mistakes riddled the federal response. Examples include: the president's lack of response to early warnings about the virus; the failure to coordinate a national supply chain for protective equipment and medication supplies, and President Trump's unwillingness to fully utilize the Defense Production Act to generate needed supplies (Shear et al., 2020). The White House also provided an ever-changing and contradictory message about COVID-19:

> The virus is not a threat; the virus is upon us. The economy must not be harmed; the economy must be shut down. There's no need to wear a mask; everyone should wear a mask – unless, like the president, you prefer not to.
> *(McManus, 2020, para. 4)*

According to Leonnig and Rucker (2021), the Trump Administration managed the pandemic as a public relations crisis rather than as an urgent national public health crisis. For example, President Trump worked to downplay the serious warnings about the pandemic that had been announced by Dr. Anthony S. Fauci, his public health adviser and the director of the National Institute of Allergy and Infectious Disease. Tension rose when Dr. Fauci remained committed to scientifically based information about the pandemic rather than minimizing its danger. As Dr. Fauci explained (McNeil, Jr., 2021: para. 9):

> We would say things like: "This is an outbreak. Infectious diseases run their own course unless one does something to intervene." And then he would get up and start talking about, "It's going to go away, it's magical, it's going to disappear."

Trump's reliance on race baiting and scapegoating worked to divert attention away from his administration's failures and alienated many Asian Americans. In March, President Trump sent two tweets referring to the "Chinese Virus." When asked about the phrasing during a White House Coronavirus briefing, Trump argued that he was merely pointing out that the illness was first detected in China (Rogers et al., 2020). His insistence on using the term further strained relations with China. In the United States, his comments immediately triggered xenophobia and increased hostility toward all Asians. As Tessler et al. noted (2020, p. 636):

> Asian Americans have historically been viewed as perpetually foreign no matter how long they have lived in the United States, therefore, it has been relatively easy for people to treat Chinese or Asian Americans as the physical embodiment of foreignness and disease.

Based on data from four U.S. cities that have large Asian-American populations (New York, San Francisco, Seattle, and Washington D.C.), Han et al. (2023) found that hate crime against Asian Americans increased significantly in 2020 compared with that in 2019. New York had the largest increase in hate crime against Asian Americans with a 3200% increase, surging from just one incident in 2019 to 33 in 2020. Furthermore, hate crime against Asian Americans temporarily spiked in March 2020 surged after terms such as "Kung flu" or "Chinese Virus" were used publicly.

Furthermore, eager to distance President Trump's reelection hopes from the pandemic's escalating death rate in the United States and the collapsing economy, the White House "[s]ought to shift responsibility for leading the fight against the pandemic to the states . . . referred to as the 'state authority handoff'" (Shear et al., 2020, para. 3). For example, to avoid responsibility for the challenges of COVID-19 testing such as the availability of test kits, President Trump argued that the CDC should have never initiated COVID-19 testing, instead, it should have been managed by the states and the private sector (Leonnig & Rucker, 2021). As Governor Cuomo (2021, p. 6) observed:

> When COVID first hit, it was inconceivable to me that the federal government would abandon its basic role of managing a federal emergency, but

> that is exactly what would happen as soon as they understood the depth of the problem, the complexity of the solution, and the political pain that needed to be endured in the coming weeks and months.

In this context, the New York State government and the City Government of New York worked to slow the spread of COVID-19 and to address critical healthcare issues (see Table 2.1). However, conflict often arose between Governor Cuomo and Mayor de Blasio over who controlled the city's plans for combatting the pandemic. This conflict did not originate in differing approaches to managing the outbreak. Instead, an ongoing feud between Governor Cuomo and Mayor de Blasio fueled division during the time of crisis (Paumgarten, 2020). In the years preceding the pandemic, Governor Cuomo often overrode de Blasio in managing city affairs, viewing the mayor as a less skilled leader. Cuomo's interventions in city management were grounded in his political philosophy that the city deferred to the power of the state and, ultimately, the power of the governor (McKinley, 2020).

Throughout the pandemic, conflicting plans were introduced by the city government and the state government, which led to confusion and heightened anxiety about the pandemic. This strife would prove deadly. On March 17, Mayor de Blasio announced the possibility of an upcoming shelter-in-place policy for city residents. Governor Cuomo immediately objected to such a policy. On March 18, Cuomo stated:

> That is not going to happen, shelter in place, for New York City. For any city or county to take an emergency action, the state has to approve it. And I wouldn't approve shelter in place. . . . Quarantine in place, you can't leave your home. The fear, the panic is a bigger problem than the virus.
>
> *(Feuer, 2020, para. 2)*

Shortly after, on March 20, Governor Cuomo finally announced that his shelter-in-place policy would begin two days later. At this point, much had already been shuttered, including educational institutions, restaurants, and entertainment venues as well as salons and gyms. However, Columbia University epidemiologists estimated that the week's delay quintupled the number of deaths in the New York metropolitan area during the first months of the pandemic (Paumgarten, 2020).

Mayor de Blasio's marginalized role in creating policy solutions to protect the city against the virus's spread differs from the great leadership roles once held by the mayors of New York during times of national crisis (Peters, 2020). For example, Mayor Rudolph W. Giuliani was praised for his powerful leadership during the September 11th crisis, earning him the title "America's Mayor."[4] In examining how Mayor Rudolph W. Giuliani's legacy was forged by his response to September 11, Powell (2007, para. 10) observes that "Political leadership is an uncertain alchemy, an admixture of the symbolic and

TABLE 2.1 New York City COVID-19 Chronology

Jan. 2020	1/11	First COVID-19 death in China
	1/21	First confirmed COVID-19 case in the United States (Washington State)
	1/30	**World Health Organization declares a global health emergency**
	1/31	President Trump bars entry of most foreign nationals who recently visited China
Feb. 2020	2/6	Cruise ship carrying passengers with COVID symptoms requests to dock in New York; Docks in New Jersey instead.
	2/29	First reported COVID-19 death in the United States (Washington State)
Mar. 2020	**3/1**	**First COVID-19 case in New York State (Manhattan)**
	3/2	Mayor de Blasio tweets that New Yorkers should ignore the virus and travel outside of city despite coronavirus
	3/3	**Second COVID-19 case in New York State (New Rochelle lawyer who worked in Manhattan)**
	3/7	Governor Andrew Cuomo declares a state of emergency
	3/8	Mayor de Blasio issues guidelines for safety: practice good hygiene, stay home if ill, telecommute, and avoid crowded subways, buses, and trains
	3/8	**16 confirmed COVID-19 cases in NYC**
	3/10	Governor Cuomo orders containment zone in New Rochelle (Lawyer from area is second COVID-19 case)
	3/11	The WHO categorizes COVID-19 outbreak as pandemic
	3/12	"Density Reduction Guidelines" issued by Governor Cuomo (events with 500+ people banned); Broadway, Museums, Concert Halls, Houses of Worship Shutter
	3/12	Mayor de Blasio declares state of emergency for city
	3/13	President Trump declares a national emergency
	3/14	**First two COVID-19 deaths in NYS**
	3/15	CDC recommends no gatherings of 50 or more people in the United States
	3/16	**NYC Public Schools Close**
	3/17	**Mayor de Blasio proposes shelter-in-place recommendation for city residents, which is overruled by Cuomo; NYC bars and restaurants shutter (delivery only)**
	3/22	**Governor Cuomo's NYS "PAUSE" order begins (shelter-in-place), all nonessential workers must stay home**
	3/25	**17,800+ COVID-19 cases in NYC, 199 fatalities**
	3/27	President signs the CARES Act
	3/27	Jacob K. Javits Center converted to field hospital
	3/27	**United States has the most COVID-19 cases in the world**
	3/28	Governor Cuomo halts all nonessential construction sites in NYS
	3/29	**30,765 confirmed COVID-19 cases, 222 COVID-19 deaths in 24-hour period (672 deaths total) in NYC**
	3/30	USNS Comfort arrives in NYC
	3/31	**Over 1,000 COVID-19 deaths in NYC**

(*Continued*)

TABLE 2.1 (Continued)

Apr. 2020	4/6	Governor Cuomo extends NYS's PAUSE order and school closures to April 29
	4/8	**Queens immigrant neighborhoods become center of NYC epicenter with 7,260 COVID-19 cases (Corona, East Elmhurst, Elmhurst, and Jackson Heights)**
	4/10	NYS reported to have more COVID-19 cases than any other country
	4/15	**Governor Cuomo orders all people to wear face masks or coverings in public places**
	4/16	Governor Cuomo extends NYS's stay-at-home order and school closures to May 15
	4/30	Governor Cuomo announces NYC subway closures from 1 a.m. to 5 a.m.
May 2020	**5/1**	**Governor Cuomo closes all schools for the remainder of the academic year**
	5/7	Governor Cuomo extends PAUSE order to June 6, but will allow counties to open by May 15 if they meet qualifications
	5/14	Governor Cuomo extends PAUSE order to May 28 for NYC and regions not meeting requirements to reopen
	5/14	**NYS State of Emergency extended to June 13**
	5/15	Governor Cuomo allows drive-in theaters, landscaping, and low-risk recreational activities to reopen
	5/23	Governor Cuomo allows gatherings of up to 10 people with social distancing
	5/27	U.S. COVID-19 deaths pass 100,000
June 2020	**6/8**	**NYC begins Phase 1 of reopening**
	6/22	NYC begins Phase 2 of reopening
	6/24	NY, NJ, and CT require travelers to self-quarantine for 14 days if traveling from hot spots
July 2020	7/6	U.S. COVID-19 deaths surpass 130,000
	7/6	NYC begins Phase 3 of reopening, without indoor dining
	719	NYC begins Phase 4 reopening, excluding malls, museums, and indoor dining/bars
	7/24	NYC reaches 227,517 COVID-19 cases and 22,934 deaths
Aug. 2020	8/4	**NYC's health commissioner (Dr. Oxiris Barbot) resigns over Mayor de Blasio's decision to assign COVID-19 testing to hospitals rather than the Department of Public Health**
Sept. 2020	9/2	Gyms in NYC reopen, but indoor group workouts and pools stay closed

(Continued)

TABLE 2.1 (Continued)

	9/8	Sheriff deputies begin stopping buses headed to Port Authority from hot spots (other states), requiring quarantine forms to be signed
	9/16	Mayor de Blasio furloughs his City Hall staff, including himself
	9/27	**Based on confusion and lack of transparency in reopening plans, the union representing NYC principals and school administrators delivers a unanimous "no confidence" vote for Mayor de Blasio and Schools Chancellor Richard Carranza**
	9/29	**Elementary students return to public school classrooms across NYC**
	9/30	Indoor dining in NYC resumes with a 25% occupancy limit
Oct 2020	10/1	NYC middle and high schools begin in-person learning
	10/2	President Donald Trump and First Lady Melania Trump test positive for coronavirus
	10/4	**Second Surge begins as COVID-19 hotspots emerge throughout the city. Mayor de Blasio announces all schools and nonessential businesses will close in nine zip codes in Brooklyn and Queens, if approved by the state**
	10/5	NYC reaches 252,000 COVID-19 cases and 23,861 deaths
	10/28	**New York reaches a half million confirmed COVID-19 cases**
Nov 2020	11/13	New COVID-19 restrictions enacted: curfews on restaurants and gyms, limited gatherings in private homes of no more than 10 people
	11/19	**NYC schools switch to all-remote**
	11/21	Renewal of indoor dining restrictions in NYC
Dec 2020	12/7	NYC public schools begin to reopen for in-person learning
	12/14	**First COVID-19 vaccination administered in the United States (Given in Queens)**
	12/21	Vaccinations begin at nursing homes
Feb 2021		**Delta Variant detected in some new COVID-19 cases**
Mar 2021		New Yorkers aged 30 and older are eligible for a vaccine; NYC high schools reopen for in-person learning
Apr 2021		New Yorkers aged 16 and up are eligible for a vaccine
Dec 2021	12/2	**NYC Health Officials confirms first 5 cases of Omicron Variant**
Mar 2022	3/6	**Mayor Adams lifts proof of vaccination to enter NYC restaurants, bars, and gyms**
	3/7	NYC Public School Students Allowed to Unmask

Source: investopedia.com, *The New York Times.*

substantive and the visceral." Speaking from downtown Manhattan shortly after the attack, Giuliani calmed the city and the nation by stating:

> Today is obviously one of the most difficult days in the history of the city. The tragedy that we are undergoing right now is something that we've had nightmares about. My heart goes out to all the innocent victims of this horrible and vicious act of terrorism. And our focus now has to be to save as many lives as possible.
>
> *(Powell, 2007, para. 6)*

In the traumatic weeks following the attack, Giuliani's resolve helped to steady the city and the nation. Mayor Giuliani was everywhere at once as he responded to the city's needs – from funerals to key city events to recovery planning sessions, offering a way for people to collectively mourn and to work together toward recovery. Later, Mayor Giuliani's shortcomings regarding the September 11th attack would be revealed.[5] Mayor La Guardia performed a similar role leading the country during crisis. In 1941, shortly before the United States entered World War II, Mayor La Guardia was appointed by President Franklin D. Roosevelt as the Head of the Office of Civilian Defense. He traveled throughout the country, encouraging Americans to prepare for war through activities such as volunteering for auxiliary units, practicing air raid drills, and learning how to shelter in place. In a speech that was later published in the *NYPD Journal*, La Guardia urged city residents to protect themselves:

> If Hitler or Hirohito feel that bombing New York City is worth the price, they will pay it. But – your city is prepared for such an attack and is ready to meet the needs of men, women and children who may be affected by it. . . . America learned the hard way that war can happen here. Your city is prepared. Are you?
>
> *(Glidden-Lyon, 2017, para. 3)*

Mayor de Blasio was not prepared for COVID-19's attack on the city. His leadership during the early months of the pandemic was viewed as "passive, reactive and inconsistent" (Peters, 2020, para. 29). Beyond tensions with Governor Cuomo, Mayor de Blasio's ineffectiveness also stemmed from his initial resistance to acknowledge the pandemic's potential impact on the city. For example, on March 11, Mayor de Blasio appeared on The Daily Show and downplayed the potential consequences of COVID-19, framing concerns as "Fear that's been generated beyond facts and reality" (Parang et al., 2020).

As a CUNY professor and as a researcher on prepping, I was shocked by Mayor de Blasio's statement. This time, The Daily Show's crazy content hit too close to home. I winced and my husband shook his head. By that time, COVID-19 had already changed my life. I had stopped traveling by early February. I was no longer riding the subway. I was already wearing an N95 mask.

I had transitioned my class to online learning. I had also begun sheltering in place. For me, the reality was clear. We were going to be hit hard. The mayor's denial generated fear and uncertainty in me. Soon enough, we were the first epicenter of COVID-19 in the United States. As the virus waged war on our city, I regularly watched de Blasio's press conferences and read his remarks in *The New York Times*, hoping for words that would ground me, mend my heart, and renew my confidence in his leadership. Those words never came. I only sensed a lack of connectedness to the city and a loss of self-assuredness. I guess I kept waiting for de Blasio to somehow repair our relationship. However, I was slow to realize that we had already broken up much earlier. In *Rolling Stone* magazine, Bort (2021) argues that Mayor de Blasio abandoned New York for his presidential bid. I agree. That's really when de Blasio broke up with the city. Mayor de Blasio seemed to fade away as Governor Cuomo's press conferences became a national platform.

The Center for Disease Control and Prevention's "COVID-19 Outbreak – New York City, February 29 – June 1, 2020" report (Thompson et al., 2020) encapsulates the effect of the pandemic's first wave: New York was the first epicenter of the COVID-19 pandemic in the United States. From March to May 2020, approximately 203,000 laboratory-confirmed COVID-19 cases were reported to the NYC Department of Health and Mental Hygiene. The overall fatality rate was 9.2% for the general population and 32.1% among those hospitalized. The first wave of COVID-19 in the city revealed that senior citizens, Black/African American and Hispanic/Latino persons, those who were living in neighborhoods with high poverty, and those with underlying medical conditions suffered disproportionately.

By early July 2020, as the number of COVID-19 cases and the number of deaths began to decline, Cuomo declared that New York had prevailed against COVID-19. In celebration of New York's victory, Cuomo released a curious graphic poster, titled "New York Tough," a mountain made in the shape of the state's COVID-19 infection curve (White, 2020) (see Figure 2.1). The poster is intended to reflect the critical time frame of the first surge – the first 111 days of the pandemic in New York (the same time span of Governor Cuomo's daily televised briefings). As Governor Cuomo explained, "We went up the mountain, we curved the mountain, we came down the other side and these are little telltale signs that, to me, represent what was going on." (July 2020). The artwork is similar to campaign posters from the early 1900s and Victorian public reform posters that utilized a collection of symbols to relay a central message (Farago, 2020). The poster was designed to depict his state's treacherous journey in overcoming the dangers and obstacles in its battle against the virus. The poster serves as both a narrative arc and a map for understanding the Governor's interpretation of how New York had worked to move to the other side of the mountain. Just like New York during those 111 days, the mountain is overwhelmed by fears, terrible events, and new rules for survival. As a bored President Trump watches from his seat on a crescent moon, threats abound, such as an airplane with the words "COVID-19" and "Europeans" written across its wings, speeding toward the mountain amid clouds labeled "FED CLOUDS of CONFUSION" and "WH TASK FORCE." Symbolizing New York's first (near) encounter with COVID-19, a cruise ship is about to be overtaken by a sea monster. The "Economy Falls" waterfall rushes downward across the mountain. Yet, the curve is pulled down by a rope held by

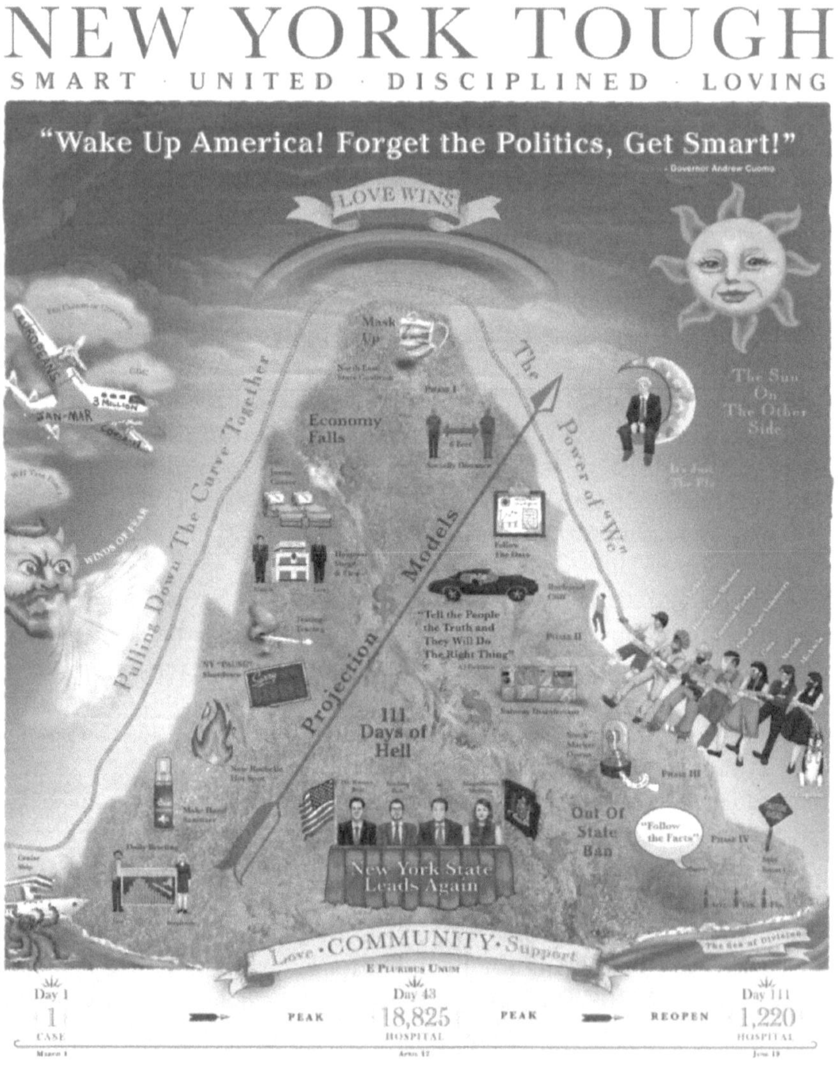

FIGURE 2.1 New York Tough Map by Gov. Andrew Cuomo.

Source: Gov. Andrew Cuomo.

dedicated mask-wearing New Yorkers (including essential workers, Cuomo's two daughters, and his dog, "Captain."[6] Jason Farago (2020, para. 12), art critic for *The New York Times*, explains, "As a work of political propaganda, this poster gets at least one job done: the federal government bears all the blame, the State of New York is diligent and triumphant."

Cuomo's poster lacks two important elements – the tragic mistake of delaying the shelter-in-place order and the nursing home tragedy. Caused by political infighting and concern over instigating panic, Governor Cuomo's delay in announcing a stay-at-home order increased the number of deaths caused by COVID-19. New York State had its first COVID-19 case on March 1; however, Governor Cuomo's order did not take effect until March 22. After determining that the timing of social distancing policies can have a powerful effect on an outbreak's death toll, epidemiologists Britta L. Jewell and Nicholas P. Jewell (2020, para. 9) found that "The growth in U.S. deaths from Covid-19 has been fueled by the devastating events in New York, where the state's stay-at-home order did not take effect until March 22." According to Dr. Thomas R. Frieden, the former head of the CDC and former commissioner of New York City's Health Department from 2007 to 2009, the state and city had adopted widespread social distancing measures a week or two earlier, including closing schools, stores, and restaurants; then the estimated death toll from the outbreak might have been reduced by 50–80% in the city (Goodman, 2020). Jewell and Jewell (2020) argue that "It is important to understand that lockdowns are not a solution to the virus, but they do buy us time to better prepare for further waves of infection and to develop treatments and vaccines."

Questions have also been raised about the cause of New York's high death rate of nursing home residents as well as the true rate of deaths. Governor Cuomo and his aides altered reports and obscured data to conceal the true number of deaths, publicly reporting 9,076 deaths (Goodman & Hakim, 2021). However, the true death toll was much higher. According to a New York State Comptroller audit, the actual death toll of nursing home residents was 15,360, with the full death toll underreported by as much as 50% from April 2020 to February 2021 (Ferre-Sadurni, 2022). Efforts to conceal these deaths by micromanaging the release of data has been viewed as evidence of Cuomo's extreme efforts to reinforce his stature as a national leader in the battle against COVID-19 (Goodman & Hakim, 2021). New York State's tragically high death rate for nursing home residents during the pandemic may have resulted from multiple factors. Governor Cuomo's state directive, which required nursing homes to readmit residents who were sent to hospitals with COVID-19 and had recovered, may have been responsible for increasing the number of deaths. Also, both mildly symptomatic and asymptomatic nursing home employees continued working throughout March and April, unknowingly spreading the virus within the facility, as the CDC was not yet aware that these individuals were contagious (Ferre-Sadurni & Harris, 2020).

The picture of Cuomo and his aides reviewing and altering documents to conceal the real death toll of nursing home residents communicates a very different message from Cuomo's poster that proclaims triumph over COVID-19. As described in *The New Yorker* (Chayka, 2020, para 5):

> The poster is reminiscent of medieval manuscript illuminations, those complicated scenes that integrate calligraphy and numerology to gesture at a truth beyond logic. The message of this latest from the atelier Cuomo is, ultimately, that we must have faith that salvation is with us. Someday we will reach "The Sun On The Other Side," whose beatific, anthropomorphized face is blessedly mask-free.

However, when Cuomo released the celebratory poster, we had not yet reached salvation. Victory was declared too early and declared falsely. After a brief lull in the summer, a second surge emerged in October 2020 and lasted through January 2021. After the first year of the pandemic, New York City had 30,303 confirmed and probable COVID-19 deaths, job losses of over 626,400, shuttered museums and cultural institutions, a dark Broadway, a 70% decrease in subway ridership, a loss of at least 187,000 households, as well as a devastated economy (King & Cole, 2021). After the second year, the city has endured over 2.3 million cases of COVID-19, including the Delta, Omicron, and BA.2 variants, which have resulted in 40,073 deaths (New York Times Coronavirus Tracking, n.d.). May 11, 2023, marked the end of the Federal COVID-19 Public Health Emergency declaration (Centers for Disease Control and Prevention, 2023).

The political context of abandonment by the federal government and turf wars between the state and local governments played a critical role in reaffirming the prepping philosophy of self-reliance. For urban preppers, the government's failure to enact a clear response to the pandemic reaffirmed their core belief: the government was not coming to save, aid, or protect them. Instead, they would need to rely on themselves and their local networks for survival. These urban preppers expressed concerns similar to other Americans about the management of the pandemic, such as the lack of presidential leadership, the shortage of protective equipment, and economic instability. It is in this context that urban preppers got to work. No, they have always been at work. Instead, they started working harder. Marlon, a seasoned prepper and the leader of the UOS, cautioned against relying on government support during the pandemic:

> Look, I said a long time ago that there was no cavalry coming. The pandemic proved that I was right in my thinking. The president, exaggerating

> claims while people are dying. Governor Cuomo and Mayor DeBlasio squabbling and holding things up while people are dying. Stop having faith in these people. We have to take care of ourselves.

As the following chapters will show, that is exactly what they did.

Notes

1 The exhibition was also supported by The Tenement Museum, New York Public Library, Brooklyn Historical Society, and the Graduate Center for the City of New York.

2 The tapestry of masks and the Styrofoam mountain were both created to be used as visual aids during Governor Cuomo's televised briefings. The tapestry was made from donated masks from Americans across the country as a sign of support for New York. Some critics argued that the masks should have been used to alleviate the mask shortage rather than made into a piece of art (Spector, 2020). The mountain was intended to represent the curve of COVID-19 cases in New York State. However, the mountain was immediately likened to Jabba the Hut and served as a source of amusement for the media and public via social media (see Bishara, 2020).

3 In comparison to Philadelphia and Boston, New York City experienced fewer deaths. New York City had an excess death rate per 1,000 was 4.7 compared to 7.3 in Philadelphia and 6.5 in Boston (Aimone, 2010). New York's strong Public Health infrastructure and policies (that had implemented to combat tuberculosis) helped reduce the number of deaths caused by the 1918 Influenza pandemic; see Aimone (2010) for a review of these public health responses.

4 However, Rudolph Giuliani experienced a fall from grace due to his role as a legal advisor and frontman for President Trump. In 2023, Giuliani was indicted along with 17 others for illegally plotting to overturn the 2020 presidential election in favor of the losing candidate, President Trump (Barry, 2023).

5 Later, the 9/11 Commission Report (2004) found that the city government's lack of preparedness could have resulted in the deaths of first responders on site after the attack. Due to faulty radio communications, many firefighters in the World Trade Center towers died because they did not hear the order to evacuate from a World Trade Center Tower. See Collins and Barrett (2009) for a critical reappraisal of Giuliani's policy decisions related to September 11 such as his 1997 decisions to locate The Office of Emergency Management to the World Trade Center rather than the recommended site in Brooklyn.

6 Captain really is not holding the rope. As the rope seems to be draped around his waist, he is more like the anchor team member in a tug-of-war.

References

Abutaleb, Y., & Paletta, D. (2021). *Nightmare scenario: Inside the Trump administration's response to the pandemic that changed history.* Harper.

Aimone, F. (2010). The 1918 influenza epidemic in New York City: A review of the public health response. *Public Health Reports, 125*(Suppl 3), 71–79.

Barry, D. (2023, August 15). From "America's Mayor" to criminal defendant: Giuliani's long tumble. *The New York Times.* www.nytimes.com/2023/08/15/nyregion/rudy-giuliani-trump-indictment.html

Bishara, H. (2020, July 1). New York governor Cuomo's COVID-19 "mountain" sculpture is as bad as it sounds. *Hyperallergic.com.* https://hyperallergic.com/574320/governor-cuomo-covid-19-mountain-sculpture/

Bort, T. (2021, April 11). Bill de Blasio burned out when New York needed him most. *Rolling Stone*. www.rollingstone.com/politics/politics-features/bill-de-blasio-new-york-city-mayor-downfall-1146337/

Brown, M. (2020, April 1). Face check: Does New York have a stockpile of thousands of unneeded ventilators? *USA Today*. www.usatoday.com/story/news/factcheck/2020/04/01/fact-check-does-new-york-have-stockpile-unneeded-ventilators/5097170002/

Calfas, J. (2020, February 7). In New Jersey, four Chinese nationals are monitored for coronavirus. *The Wall Street Journal*. www.wsj.com/articles/in-new-jersey-four-chinese-nationals-are-monitored-for-coronavirus-11581106998

Centers for Disease Control and Prevention. (2023, September 27). *What ending the COVID-19 public health emergency means for you*. www.cdc.gov/coronavirus/2019-ncov/your-health/end-of-phe.html

Chayka, K. (2020, July 16). Andrew Cuomo's pandemic poster and the limits of coronavirus visuals. *The New Yorker*. www.newyorker.com/culture/dept-of-design/andrew-cuomos-pandemic-poster-and-the-limits-of-coronavirus-visual

Collins, D., & Barrett, W. (2009). *Grand illusion: The untold story of Rudy Giuliani and 9/11*. HarperCollins e-books.

Cuomo, A. (2020a). *American crisis: Leadership lessons from the COVID-19 pandemic*. Crown.

Cuomo, A. (2020b, July 13). New York tough poster. *New York State*. www.governor.ny.gov/new-york-tough-poster

Cuomo, A. (2020c, July 13). Video, photos, audio & rush transcript: Governor Cuomo announces new data-driven guidance for reopening schools. *Governor of New York*. www.governor.ny.gov/news/video-photos-audio-rush-transcript-governor-cuomo-announces-new-data-driven-guidance-reopening

Cuomo, A. (2020d, March 24). Video, audio, photos & rush transcript: Governor Cuomo: In New York, "love wins and it will win again through this virus". *Governor of New York*. www.governor.ny.gov/news/video-audio-photos-rush-transcript-governor-cuomo-new-york-love-wins-and-it-will-win-again

Druckman, B., & Young, M. (2021, February 23). New exhibit germ city at the Museum of the City of New York explores disease and the metropolis. *Untapped New York*. https://untappedcities.com/2018/09/14/new-exhibit-germ-city-at-the-museum-of-the-city-of-new-york-explores-disease-and-the-metropolis/

Dwyer, C. (2020, November 21). Andrew Cuomo to receive international Emmy for "masterful" COVID-19 briefings. *NPR*. www.npr.org/sections/coronavirus-live-updates/2020/11/21/937445923/andrew-cuomo-to-receive-international-emmy-for-masterful-covid-19-briefings

Farago, J. (2020, July 14). Andrew Cuomo ascends to the mountaintop with his pandemic poster. *The New York Times*. www.nytimes.com/2020/07/14/arts/design/cuomo-covid-poster-new-york.html

Faust, J. S., Lin, Z., & Del Rio, C. (2020). Comparison of estimated excess deaths in New York City during the COVID-19 and 1918 influenza pandemics. *JAMA Network Open*, *3*(8), e2017527–e2017527.

Ferré-Sadurní, L. (2022, March 15). Health agency under Cuomo "misled the public" on nursing home deaths. *The New York Times*. www.nytimes.com/2022/03/15/nyregion/nursing-home-deaths-cuomo-covid.html

Ferré-Sadurní, L., & Harris, A. (2020, July 8). Does Cuomo share blame for 6,200 virus deaths in N.Y. nursing homes? *The New York Times*. www.nytimes.com/2020/07/08/nyregion/nursing-homes-deaths-coronavirus.html

Feuer, W. (2020, March 18). Gov. Cuomo says he won't approve coronavirus "shelter-in-place" order for New York City after mayor tells residents to prepare. *CNBC*. www.cnbc.com/2020/03/18/cuomo-says-he-wont-approve-coronavirus-shelter-in-place-order-for-new-york-city.html

Glidden-Lyon, S. (2017, November 16). This is no clam bake: Mayor La Guardia and the office of civilian defense. *NYC Department of Records & Information Services*. www.archives.nyc/blog/2017/11/16/laguardia-and-civil-defense
Goldstein, J., & McKinley, J. (2020, March 2). Coronavirus in N.Y.: Manhattan woman is first confirmed case in state. *The New York Times*. www.nytimes.com/2020/03/01/nyregion/new-york-coronvirus-confirmed.html
Goodman, D., & Hakim, D. (2021, March 4). Cuomo aides rewrote nursing home report to hide higher death toll. *The New York Times*. www.nytimes.com/2021/03/04/nyregion/cuomo-nursing-home-deaths.html
Goodman, J. (2020, April 8). How delays and unheeded warnings hindered New York's virus fight. *The New York Times*. www.nytimes.com/2020/04/08/nyregion/new-york-coronavirus-response-delays.html
Gordon, B. (2020). *Life after COVID-19: Lessons from past pandemics*. Banovallum Books.
Han, S., Riddell, J. R., & Piquero, A. R. (2023). Anti-Asian American hate crimes spike during the early stages of the COVID-19 pandemic. *Journal of Interpersonal Violence*, *38*(3–4), 3513–3533.
Hartocollis, A. (2009, June 10). 12 flu victims have died, and ill may total 550,000. *The New York Times*. www.nytimes.com/2009/06/11/nyregion/11flu.html
Hartocollis, A. (2009, May 17). New York reports its first Swine Flu death. *The New York Times*. www.nytimes.com/2009/05/18/nyregion/18swine.html
Ijeoma, E. (2018). *Pan-African AIDS*. https://studioijeoma.com/Pan-African-AIDS
Jewell, B., & Jewell, H. (2020, April 14). The huge cost of waiting to contain the pandemic. *The New York Times*. www.nytimes.com/2020/04/14/opinion/covid-social-distancing.html
King, K., & Cole, D. (2021, March 16). How a year of the COVID-19 pandemic changed New York City. The numbers are in. *The Wall Street Journal*. www.wsj.com/story/the-numbers-are-in-how-a-year-of-the-covid-19-pandemic-changed-new-york-city-60251164
Leonnig, C., & Rucker, P. (2021). *I alone can fix It: Donald J. Trump's catastrophic final year*. Penguin Publishing Group.
Lewis, R. (2020, March 30). New York's existing plans for pandemics were not enough for the current crisis. *City & State New York*. www.cityandstateny.com/policy/2020/03/new-yorks-existing-plans-for-pandemics-were-not-enough-for-the-current-crisis/176178/
McKinley, J. (2020, January 9). Cuomo's 2020 vision: Turbulent waters and so many octopuses. *The New York Times*. www.nytimes.com/2020/01/09/nyregion/2020-cuomo-poster-ny.html
McManus, D. (2020, April 8). Column: Trump's "I'm not responsible" presidency. *Los Angeles Times*. www.latimes.com/politics/story/2020-04-08/trumps-im-not-responsible-presidency
McNeil, D. (2021, January 24). Fauci on what working for Trump was really like. *The New York Times*. www.nytimes.com/2021/01/24/health/fauci-trump-covid.html
Moores, K. (2018, June 11). Wellcome launches Contagious Cities. *Press Release*. https://wellcome.org/press-release/wellcome-launches-contagious-cities
Museum of the City of New York. (2018). Germ city: Microbes and the Metropolis. *Museum of the City of New York*. www.mcny.org/exhibition/germ-city
National Commission on Terrorist Attacks Upon the United States. (2004). *The 9/11 commission report*. http://govinfo.library.unt.edu/911/report/911Report.pdf
New York City Department of Health. (2019). *Zika virus*. https://www1.nyc.gov/site/doh/health/health-topics/zika-virus.page
New York Times. (n.d.). Tracking coronavirus in New York: latest map and case count. *The New York Times*. www.nytimes.com/interactive/2021/us/new-york-covid-cases.html

Nir, S. M., & Mckinley, J. (2020, March 10). "Containment area" is ordered for New Rochelle coronavirus cluster. *The New York Times*. www.nytimes.com/2020/03/10/nyregion/coronavirus-new-rochelle-containment-area.html
Parang, C. (Writer), Amira, D. (Writer), & Pennolino, P. (Director). (2020, March 11). Bill de Blasio & Lil' Dicky (Season 33, Episode 87) [TV series episode]. In T. Noah, J. Katz, & J. Flanz (Executive Producers), *The daily show with Trevor Noah*. Ark Angel; Comedy Partners Film Productions.
Paumgarten, P. (2020, June 17). Andrew Cuomo, the king of New York. *The New Yorker*. www.newyorker.com/magazine/2020/10/19/andrew-cuomo-the-king-of-new-york
Peters, J. (2020, April 8). Trump and de Blasio: "Together, at the wrong time in history". *The New York Times*. www.nytimes.com/2020/06/17/us/politics/trump-bill-de-blasio-new-york.html
Port Authority NY-NJ. (2020). Port authority airports and road and rail network report record passenger and cargo volumes for 2019. *The Port Authority of New York and New Jersey*. www.panynj.gov/port-authority/en/press-room/press-release-archives/2020-press-releases/port-authority-airports-and-road-and-rail-network-report-record-.html
Powell, M. (2007, September 21). In 9/11 chaos, Giuliani forged a lasting image. *The New York Times*. www.nytimes.com/2007/09/21/us/politics/21giuliani.html
Rogers, J. P., Chesney, E., Oliver, D., Pollak, T. A., McGuire, P., Fusar-Poli, P., Zandi, M. S., Lewis, G., & David, A. S. (2020). Psychiatric and neuropsychiatric presentations associated with severe coronavirus infections: A systematic review and meta-analysis with comparison to the COVID-19 pandemic. *Lancet Psychology*, 7(7), 611–627.
Rosen, C. (2020, November 24). Andrew Cuomo accepts Emmy award as coronavirus cases continue to rise. *Vanity Fair*. www.vanityfair.com/hollywood/2020/11/andrew-cuomo-emmy-award
Rosenthal, B., Pinkowski, J., & Goldstein, J. (2020, March 26). "The other option is death": New York starts sharing of ventilators. *The New York Times*. www.nytimes.com/2020/03/26/health/coronavirus-ventilator-sharing.html
Sanger, D., Kanno-Youngs, Z., & Kulish, N. (2020, April 1). A ventilator stockpile, with one hitch: Thousands do not work. *The New York Times*. www.nytimes.com/2020/04/01/us/politics/coronavirus-ventilators.html
Santora, M. (2014). First patient quarantined under strict new policy tests negative for Ebola. *The New York Times*. www.nytimes.com/2014/10/25/nyregion/new-york-ebola-case-craig-spencer.html?searchResultPosition=3
Shear, M. D., Weiland, N., Lipton, E., Haberman, M., & Sanger, D. E. (2020, July 28). Inside Trump's failure: The rush to abandon leadership role on the virus. *The New York Times*. www.nytimes.com/2020/07/18/us/politics/trump-coronavirus-response-failure-leadership.html
Slavitt, A. (2021). *Preventable: The inside story of how leadership failures, politics, and selfishness doomed the U.S. coronavirus response*. St. Martin's Publishing Group.
Spector, J. (2020, April 29). Gov. Andrew Cuomo shows a mural of donated masks to New York. Then social media weighed in. *Times Herald-Record*. www.recordonline.com/story/news/2020/04/29/gov-andrew-cuomo-shows-mural-of-donated-masks-to-new-york-then-social-media-weighed-in/111717324/
Tessler, H., Choi, M., & Kao, G. (2020). The anxiety of being Asian American: Hate crimes and negative biases during the COVID-19 pandemic. *American Journal of Criminal Justice*, *45*(4), 636–646.
Thompson, C. N., Baumgartner, J., Pichardo, C., et al. (2020). COVID-19 outbreak – New York City, February 29 – June 1, 2020. *Morbidity and Mortality Weekly Report*, *69*, 1725–1729. http://doi.org/10.15585/mmwr.mm6946a2

Weissman Center for International Business, Baruch College/CUNY. (2010). NYC data [Data set]. In *New York City (NYC) Yellow Fever Epidemic – 1795 to 1804*. www.baruch.cuny.edu/nycdata/disasters/yellow_fever.html

White, K. (2020, July 15). We decoded the symbols in New York governor Andrew Cuomo's bizarre new pandemic poster, from "boyfriend cliff" to that sinister octopus. *Artnet News*. https://news.artnet.com/art-world/cuomo-pandemic-poster-decoded-1894782

Winegard, T. C. (2020). *The mosquito: A human history of our deadliest predator*. Dutton Books.

Zimmer, C. (2020, April 9). Most New York coronavirus cases came from Europe, genomes show. *The New York Times*. www.nytimes.com/2020/04/08/science/new-york-coronavirus-cases-europe-genomes.html

3

ESCAPE FROM NEW YORK

When the Rich Left the City

To understand the story of the mass exodus of the wealthy from New York City to escape COVID-19 is to understand that it is not entirely a new story. The rich have always escaped cities during pandemics. At its core, the story is also another reflection of the sharp division between classes in New York and between the way they know the world. In an *Atlantic* article titled, "Affluence Killed New York, Not the Pandemic," Baker (2020) argues that New York has become overly dependent on the whims of the very wealthy, transforming the city into a place for the superrich rather than a safe and affordable city for working people. As Baker (2020) observes, "the city is in the midst of a reckoning – not simply because of the coronavirus, but because of what it had already become."

It is also not just one, but many stories about the consequences of the flight of the rich from the city at the start of the pandemic. There are also many storytellers. As a sociologist, my intention is to share a complex and comprehensive narrative that helps the readers grasp the powerful interconnections between the structural and the personal. This is a story of the consequences and layers of resentment, based mostly on economics and geography. While the exodus of the wealthy had a detrimental effect on the city, the arrival of the rich at their hideaways also negatively impacted many of those areas. Wealthy New Yorkers viewed their respective destinations as a refuge, whereas local residents of these communities sometimes viewed these New Yorkers as intruders. In the city that the wealthy had abandoned, residents resented the abandonment of neighborhoods and the subsequent diminished tax base. In the new locales, residents resented their neighborhoods being overtaken and consumed by the city's relocated wealthy. In turn, the rich resented being resented in both places. In response to a *New York Times* article about the

DOI: 10.4324/9781003400356-3

wealthy leaving the city (Quealy, 2020), one reader posted the epigraph from the novel *Appointment in Samarra* (O'Hara, 1934) as a reminder that the rich may not be able to escape their fates. (Death is the epigraph's narrator.):

> There was a merchant in Baghdad who sent his servant to market to buy provisions and in a little while the servant came back, white and trembling, and said, Master, just now when I was in the marketplace I was jostled by a woman in the crowd and when I turned I saw it was Death that jostled me. She looked at me and made a threatening gesture, now, lend me your horse, and I will ride away from this city and avoid my fate. I will go to Samarra and there Death will not find me. The merchant lent him his horse, and the servant mounted it, and he dug his spurs in its flanks and as fast as the horse could gallop he went. Then the merchant went down to the marketplace and he saw me standing in the crowd and he came to me and said, Why did you make a threating gesture to my servant when you saw him this morning? That was not a threatening gesture, I said, it was only a start of surprise. I was astonished to see him in Bagdad, for I had an appointment with him tonight in Samarra.

Yet, this story is not only about resentment. It is also about heartbreak. For many who left the city, their departure may have been quick, but that did not mean that it was without anguish. My memories of the tears and goodbyes in the lobby of my Greenwich apartment building are reminiscent of this. At the beginning of February 2020, the floor of my building had 16 occupied apartments. Tenants ranged from a family with four young children (The preschooler loved to belt out Lady Gaga's "Bad Romance") to an elegant manager who had fresh flowers delivered weekly to her apartment with an all-white decor, to an incredibly fun single financial analyst whose living room closely resembled an Irish pub, to an engaged couple who owned an irresistible, too-energetic Bernese-Doodle puppy. By June, my floor had only three occupied apartments.

The puppy and his sweet owners left first. I felt for them. They were poised to begin their life together in the city. Instead, COVID-19 had cheated them of that pleasure. They were forced to cancel their March wedding and had decided to return home until the pandemic ended. They never returned. The financial analyst left next. Carrying his golf clubs, he mumbled something about taking an extended vacation as we shared an elevator ride. Sheltering-in-place had one saving grace. I was almost able to avoid the awkwardness of the other move-outs. However, a neighbor in the building frequently updated me on those who were moving out. Our conversations always ended the same way – with an assessment of whether the person was still a real New Yorker. They usually weren't. Real New Yorkers stuck it out. While I did not share my friend's resentment, I did understand its origins.

In *Bracing for the Apocalypse*, I discussed how, in response to a disaster, the retreat of extremely wealthy NYC preppers to secret destinations or to safe rooms would work to undermine democracy. I argued that, by leaving the city, these high-net-worth (HNW) preppers would be withdrawing from a shared experience and opting out of working for the collective good. My argument was sound. However, the danger of this withdrawal was greater than I had anticipated. Given the advance warning of the pandemic, the HNW preppers were not the only wealthy New Yorkers to leave the city. Instead, this subgroup was joined by roughly 420,000 other rich New Yorkers. Like the HNW preppers, many of the city's wealthy residents chose to "bug out," to leave the city for a safe haven (a predetermined location or a place away from the disaster area). While their exodus was not as fully planned as the HNW preppers, it was similar. New York's rich quickly adopted the prepper's approach to bugging out: identifying a safe haven (such as a second home or vacation town), planning a route to get there (swiftly leaving the city to limit exposure), securing emergency provisions (ensuring that their safe havens had ample food and supplies), and adapting to changing circumstances (using their wealth to address unanticipated needs). In short, their wealth allowed greater flexibility. They were able to pivot with great ease, as they escaped the city to hunker down in an area for an indeterminate length of time. According to Rushkoff (2023), their extreme wealth and privilege allows them to both insulate themselves against danger and to escape from the rest of us.

This chapter analyzes the narratives surrounding the rich's abandonment of New York during the pandemic. Exploring the real and feared consequences offers insight into how this exodus represents the ever-increasing polarization between classes in the city. Perspectives on this issue from New Yorkers who remained in the city during the pandemic will be shared to study the cultural significance of wealthy residents' departure (and delayed return) to the city such as fears of white flight and an impending financial crisis. The next section discusses the significant pressure that their relocation had on their new homes as New York's wealthy shifted from temporary visitors to permanent residents, creating soaring housing prices, congestion, demands on health care and food supplies, and school systems that were overwhelmed. The chapter closes by arguing that the departure from the city by the extremely wealthy and their seamless relocation to safe havens reflects the inequality of "the velvet rope economy" that has allowed America's rich to glide past the dangers and inconveniences endured by ordinary Americans (Schwartz, 2020).

As early as mid-March, the plans of the rich to bug out of the city were clear and already underway. A *New York Times* article reminded readers that

> Broad-scale emergencies never fail to reveal the fault lines in the American class system, and it was suddenly clear that well-off New Yorkers were going to go about the business of combating the coronavirus differently, with

> more than fortitude and Purell, because they had a powerful inoculant: secondary real estate.
>
> *(Bellafante, 2020)*

Leaving the city offered several advantages for these city dwellers. First, by relocating outside New York, individuals were able to avoid the risk of transmission in a densely populated urban center. This risk was significant as New York would become the country's first epicenter. Practicing social distance would be easier in areas with smaller populations that were more spread out and where most people resided in single-family homes rather than apartments. Residing in a single-family dwelling offered the critical advantage of more interior and exterior space. Working from home was much easier with more space for setting up new home offices or utilizing those that already existed. This advantage was critical as many high tech and professional positions quickly transitioned to working virtually. Additional rooms could also be used for virtual learning and study spaces for students. Furthermore, the extra room could also be used as guest spaces for older relatives or friends who lived alone. Single-family dwellings also provided outdoor space, often with play equipment, pools, and outdoor barbecues. Both adults and children could enjoy outdoor activities rather than remaining confined to an apartment. Access to the outdoors permitted a sense of freedom and the ability "to blow off steam," which benefited mental health. Some areas also offered outdoor spaces such as the beach and hiking trails for additional enjoyment, sometimes even enjoyed when closed. As Coven and Gupta (2020, p. 3) note,

> the flexibility to work remotely allows individuals to limit outdoor physical presence and more readily leave the city to shelter with friends and family, second homes provide protective insurance against continued presence in the city, and access to additional delivery options may improve adherence to stay-in-place orders.

According to *The New York Times* analysis of three studies of aggregated smartphone location data, nearly 5% of residents, or about 420,000 people, left the city between March 1 and May 1 (Quealy, 2020).[1] The residents who left the city were overwhelming from New York's richest neighborhoods, mainly in Manhattan. The residential populations of wealthy neighborhoods such as the Upper East Side, Soho, the West Village, and Brooklyn Heights dropped by 40% due to the pandemic. Conversely, neighborhoods with median household incomes of $90,000 or less lost few residents. The profile of New York neighborhoods where more than 25% of residents left the city reflects the sharp inequality within the city (Quealy, 2020). These wealthy enclaves differ greatly from other city neighborhoods. They have higher rents and lower poverty rates. The majority of residents are White and college educated in contrast to other neighborhoods. The household income within these neighborhoods is substantially higher than the $60,521 median income in other parts of the city. More than half of the residents of these neighborhoods have a household income over $100,000 with one in three households earning more than $200,000. As reported by Coven and Gupta (2020), Manhattan residents and residents of wealthy sections of Brooklyn were much more likely to leave the city due to the pandemic, whereas resident of Queens, the epicenter of COVID-19 in the city, as well as most Brooklyn residents and those in the Bronx were substantially more likely to remain. Staten Island did not experience a significant population loss during the first months of the pandemic. As a stronghold for Trump and the Republican party, some Staten Island residents resisted policies designed to slow the spread of COVID, perceiving the measures as too restrictive (Fitzsimmons & Petri, 2020).[2]

New York City residents with the ability to leave usually went where they had pre-existing social networks and could be close to family and friends (Coven & Gupta, 2020). Wealthy New Yorkers relocated mainly to areas surrounding the city, such as Long Island's Nassau and Suffolk counties, Pennsylvania's Monroe County, New Jersey's Monmouth County, Westchester County, Connecticut's Fairfield County, and panned out farther in all directions to places like the Catskills region (Quealy, 2020). The relocation map includes popular vacation towns for second homes like The Hamptons, the Pocono Mountains, the Jersey Shore, the Catskill Mountains, and the affluent suburbs of Westchester and Fairfield. Palm Beach was also a popular destination. As wealthy New Yorkers began to relocate to these areas, year-round residents grew concerned that the influx of people from New York City would cause an increase in demand for critical services and goods. In addition, there was a concern that these escapees from the center of infections at the time would bring the virus with them. A year-round Hamptons resident pointed out the primary issue: "The biggest problem – what really gets me going – is that they think because they're all the way out [here], they're safe," says Katsipis. "But some of those people are sick, and they're going out to bars and acting like they're on vacation. What do these city people think – we have some imaginary, magical bubble?" (Gould, 2020). Locals feared that their medical care systems, food supplies, and police forces would be overwhelmed. As the mayor of Long Beach Township, NJ, Joseph Mancini explained, "We love the summer people, they drive our economy. But when they come down here now, the services here aren't geared up for them" (Tully & Stowe, 2020).

Backlash against visitors in these areas ranged from angry social media posts to warnings from local government officials to the actual barricading of some towns (Tully & Stowe, 2020). In late March 2020, three Hudson Valley counties north of the city, Greene, Delaware, and Sullivan, familiar with the additional pressures of seasonal residents and visitors during the summer, issued statements that urged the residents of New York City to stay in their primary homes (Burton, 2020). Sullivan County Public Health Director Nancy McGraw explained that "[their] message was a plea to consider the ramifications and resources before leaving one community for another" (Burton, 2020). Sullivan County has only one hospital with two locations and a food supply system unable to meet the demands of a surge in population. On its county website, Greene County cautioned that travel "from any area that this time is inadvisable and is highly discouraged" (Tully & Stowe, 2020). The "Mountain Top" area of Greene County, where the majority of second homes are located, lacks a hospital and has only two physicians (Burton, 2020). To prevent empty shelves, local grocery stores sometimes worked to limit the quantity or weight of items purchased to ensure availability to all customers rather than permitting wealthy customers to purchase everything. For example, local grocery stores in places like Woodstock in New York's Ulster County posted signs indicating quantity limits or discussed restrictions with customers if needed (such as, at the butcher counter, reminding customers to leave meat for other customers). However, shopping in the Hamptons was less genteel as newcomers ransacked stores by buying large quantities of expensive goods such as salmon, steak, and rare wines, with one customer spending more than $8,000 (Gould, 2020). According to Joe Gurrera, the manager of Citarella, a gourmet grocery store in the Hamptons:

> Instead of asking for one or two steaks on a tray, a customer will buy the whole tray. Then they'll move on to shrimp, and buy all the shrimp, and then they'll buy all the salmon steaks. . . . Instead of asking for a slice of lasagna, they'll buy all of it. Then they'll buy all of our root vegetables.
>
> *(Gould, 2020)*

Locals from the vacation towns were right about the spread of the virus. City dwellers not only hastened the spread of COVID-19, but on a much larger scale that exceeded the boundaries of their small towns. By early March, the COVID-19 outbreak in New York City was so extensive that the city became the primary site of new infections in the United States as thousands of infected people traveled from the city and sparked outbreaks throughout the country (Carey & Glanz, 2020). Travelers who helped spread the virus included New York residents who left the city and non-New Yorkers who visited or passed through the city. Tracking signature mutations of the virus, examining travel histories of infected people, and studying models of the outbreak revealed that infections spreading from New York accounted for 60% to 65% of the sequenced viruses across the country. As an international gateway, New York's immense outbreak was partly fueled by the volume of passengers to and from Europe. By the time the federal government had blocked most visitors from Europe and stay-at-home orders were issued, the virus had already spread across the country.

As the city's COVID-19 infection rate rapidly increased, governors of other states asked New York residents to stay away or imposed 14-day quarantine for visitors from the city. By the end of March 2020, governors of states such as Florida, Hawaii, Alaska, Rhode Island, South Carolina, and the territory of Puerto Rico had moved to impose these restrictions (Mazzei et al., 2020). The governors argued that the long-term benefits of trying to avoid an increase in the number of COVID-19 cases outweighed the boost of tourist dollars spent in their respective states. Governor Ron DeSantis of Florida, a Republican, signed an executive order requiring a 14-day quarantine of anyone who had arrived from the New York since the start of the month. Furthermore, all new arrivals were required to report the names of people they have had contact with to public health officials for tracing (Mazzei et al., 2020). Governor DeSantis argued that "Maybe they haven't even shown symptoms, but they could be infected. After all the hard work, we don't want it to now get seeded as people flee the hot zone" (Mazzei et al., 2020).

For the HNW prepper, bugging out practices include the purchase of a secret strategic relocation destination (a retreat for survival), which may be located in exotic locales, remote areas, or second homes. Gaston Bachelard once wrote, "If I were asked to name the chief benefit of a house, I should say that: the house shelters day dreaming, the house protects the dreamer, the house allows one to dream in peace" (1958, p. 28). Searching for a strategic relocation might be thought of as house-hunting for how the buyer dreams about the end of days. Strategic relocation is a process that involves finding an area with strong long-term security from man-made or natural threats (Skousen & Skousen, 2011). It calls for assessing the continuing safety of a place based on criteria such as geography and climate, crime rate and standard of living, government stability, and the likelihood of terrorism or war. In addition to climate and government stability, a suitable location also includes a high quality of life. Personal preference and familiarity are also important factors.

Greg, a HNW prepper who usually lives in Manhattan, owns a strategic relocation that also functions as his family's beach house in a private coastal community in the South. I toured Greg's strategic relocation when writing my first book on urban preppers. Greg works in the financial sector. This middle-aged prepper invested in a strategic location because, after the extended Occupy Wall Street protests, he became concerned about social upheaval and rioting. Set back a few blocks from the ocean on a large lot, the family's stunning and expansive beach home is built to be resilient against hurricanes. The house windows could be shuttered quickly to protect its occupants against both hurricanes and intruders. On an upper floor, an oversized family room was outfitted with items like a large, well-stocked gun cabinet, a walk-in prepper closet (including food, medicine and other supplies such as high-end binoculars and two drones). In beach houses, upper floors are viewed as important real estate because they are comparatively safe during floods. The family room/prepping room's location suggests that it is significant to the family. Greg explained that his family left the city in early February to avoid having to face any challenges such as travel restrictions. His goal was for his family to be already residing in their safe haven to avoid any anxiety about their relocation. As he explained:

> I followed my plan, a take on the Gray Man approach. In the event of a pandemic, I knew that there would be absolutely no question that New York was going to be hit hard. My plan was to leave immediately so that we would already be living here before any resistance arose about the arrival of outsiders. The transition was quiet and seamless. I planned for this. No rushing about for us by our property manager. Our pantry and freezers are always well stocked. From clothes to cars, we had everything waiting for us. We had medical supplies and my gun cabinet, if needed. My wife and I arrived first. Next, our children came home after their colleges moved online (Of course, no one took notice as their own kids were returning home, too). As I expected, fear increased and then came talk of restrictions. Owners started complaining about New Yorkers and people from New Jersey bringing the virus with them (Never mind that many of these owners are from these two states). Home rentals to New Yorkers and those from New Jersey were then banned. By that time, we had been living here for nearly two months.

I also received an encrypted note from another HNW prepper (who chooses to remain anonymous) in late February. His note read "Wishing you health and safety. Hope that you leave the city. In Wyoming for duration. Good Luck." Again, I first interviewed this prepper before the pandemic. At a Greenwich village coffee shop, he recognized me from a short *Wall Street Journal* article that discussed my project and featured a photo of me. He introduced himself and suggested that we "compare notes about prepping." He has always been personable and insightful during our discussions. However, like many wealthy preppers, he views preparedness as an extension of risk management. When thinking about disaster, preppers of ordinary means tend to focus mainly on saving people, but those with greater wealth have broader considerations. His preparedness formula is different. His plans include protecting both his people and his portfolio.

After fleeing to the Hamptons in March, many city residents decided to make the area their permanent home.[3] As the pandemic dragged on, many decided to buy a home instead of spending thousands of dollars on a summer rental. Prompted by low interest rates and virtual meeting technology that made working from home possible, some city transplants enrolled their children in local public and private schools, which has changed the affluent weekend and summer getaway into a year-round community (Sussman Fischler, 2021).

For Hamptons real estate, 2020 was a record-breaking year for the prices and the number of sales. According to the Brown Harris Stevens (2021) annual market report for 2020, the total dollar volume for 2020 was 79% as compared to 2019, with a historic high of $5.89 billion, which beat the previous record of $4.42 billion set in 2014. Furthermore, the total number of sales in the Hamptons increased by 44.1%, with 2,508 sales in 2020, compared to 1,741 in 2019. This represents the highest number of yearly sales in 15 years. Due to the high demand and limited inventory, both the average and median prices reached record highs in 2020, with sales prices in the Hamptons averaging $2.35 million, 24.2% higher than in 2019, and an all-time high for the year-end average price. The median price increased by 35.7% to $1.35 million, another record high and the first time the year-end median price exceeded the million-dollar threshold. For the first quarter of 2021, home sales in the Hamptons increased again, up 48% compared to the historic high of 2020 (Bernstein, 2021b).

In contrast, the pandemic caused the city's luxury real estate market to plummet faster than the declines brought on by both the 2008 financial crisis and the 9/11 terrorist attacks. Between March and August 2020, overall sales of Manhattan homes were down 56%. For properties priced at $4 million or higher, sales were down 67% (Clarke, 2020). Manhattan's apartment rental market also tumbled. By fall 2020, apartment listings in the city's wealthiest borough had tripled from 2019, to 15,923, the highest inventory rate on record (Carmiel, 2020). In August 2020, the Douglas Elliman's Real Estate (2021) report for Manhattan reflected the uncharacteristically weak market for rentals:

> There was the largest market share of landlord concessions in nearly a decade of tracking and the highest total of listing inventory in over fourteen years and the third straight monthly record. The vacancy rate exceeds 5% for the first time and the fourth consecutive month with a new record.

With Manhattan's offices, cultural institutions, restaurants, and fashionable stores all shuttered, the city's appeal had vanished, at least temporarily.

As the pandemic dragged on, tensions and public debate about those who left the city continued. For Jeremiah Moss, author of *Vanishing New York*, a book and a blog about the negative impact of gentrification on New York culture, his resentment toward those who left the city is not directed toward

> the ones who departed because of lost jobs, underlying illness or the need to take care of aged parents; instead, [it was meant for] the large group of

> people who left because they didn't know how to be in New York without consuming, without being in bars and restaurants and stores.
>
> *(Bernstein, 2021a)*

For those who remained, staying in the city was perceived as a display of courage and dedication to New York. However, class-based resentment toward those who could afford to leave remains clear. The reflections of one Harlem resident who stayed in the city illustrate this complex mix of resentment and resiliency:

> Those who were able to go away don't understand that how we survive in the city is a tremendously high-pressure situation. We, those who left and those who stayed, have the same limited knowledge about the virus but our level of fear is very different. My husband and I take a walk in the park every two weeks, wearing masks and gloves. People who went to Connecticut and those who went other places, they do it all, sit outside, take walks, hike, and all without masks. For us, everything is a risk. Now, we know how strong we are.

According to a Manhattan therapist who met virtually with patients throughout the pandemic:

> Tensions that were always there were intensified. Wealth afforded all sorts of protection for some New Yorkers, like the luxury of being able to escape to a second home. Without means, many who stayed in the city felt less protected and more vulnerable. However, class division only represents one rift. There was tension among the affluent due to differences in professions. Service vs. Escape. There were those who chose to continue working at hospitals or participated in other ways to help when they could have left. They were disappointed by the decision of others to just flee.

Guilt did seem to emerge among some New Yorkers who left the city. In a *New York Times* Op-Ed article titled, "I Left My Troubled City Behind. Now I Feel Guilty," journalist George Blecher (2020) discussed the sadness of leaving New York as someone who was at high risk:

> I knew that I was joining the exodus of the privileged. I've also felt guilty. Not about finding a safe shelter – as far as I can see, it was the wisest move for all concerned – but about having to leave my friends and neighbors.

Beyond leaving friends and family during the pandemic, some New Yorkers also missed New York's cultural and creative energy. A *New York Times* study found that some city transplants were actually seeking to find an approximate of New York. Between July 2020 and July 2021, some relocated New Yorkers searching for homes in nine major metro areas predominantly looked in urban and downtown neighborhoods, prioritizing public transportation and the availability of short-term leases, perhaps leaving open the chance to return home (Miller, 2020). However, some New Yorkers felt no regrets about fleeing the city to protect their families. As one anonymous New Yorker who took refuge with her family in a second home outside of the city said:

> I don't begrudge feeling a little bit like you've earned some sort of Girl Scout or Boy Scout badge because you've been through something. I'm not going to put my family's health at risk when I have the option not to. . . . If you want to win the true New Yorker contest, go for it. You win.
>
> *(Ruiz, 2020b)*

The public debate regarding the exodus of the rich from New York is significant because it is a stark reminder of the sharp class divisions in this global capital. New York City has one of the highest rates of income disparity in the nation (Bach, 2020). The wealthy's willingness to buy its escape from the pandemic is a powerful example of the Velvet Rope Economy, "a Versailles-like world of pampering for a privileged few on one side of the velvet rope, a mad scramble for basic service for everyone else" (Schwartz, 2020, p. 2). However, class-based resentment may not be the only explanation for the backlash against the wealthy leaving the city. Instead, this resentment also seems to stem from their decision to break with a perceived social contract with other New Yorkers and to reject the shared experiences of enduring the pandemic together as city dwellers. As the Manhattan therapist further explains, "those who experienced the pandemic together in the city formed a special bond, an understanding of what it was like to hold steady in tight quarters when tractor-trailers, operating as morgues, were parked on the streets." As an antithesis of urban citizenship, the mass exodus rejected the local and the possibilities of the city. The mass exodus seemed to undermine the belief in the collective spirit's ability to overcome adversity. It represented pulling away rather than pulling together.

While the mass exodus of the rich from New York does reflect class division, this single narrative does have weaknesses. The narrative of those who left the city as self-absorbed and insensitive is inaccurate. Leaving the city, leaving one's identity, was not an easy decision for many individuals (particularly those who moved permanently – unlike the temporary transplants who had a second home). For many city dwellers, the identity of being a New Yorker was closely connected to one's decision to stay or leave during the pandemic. In March 2020, a Facebook group called "Into the Unknown" was formed for New Yorkers who had made the decision to leave, or who were debating leaving the city. With over 14,000 members, this private

Facebook group served as a discussion group and information resource for "those of us who have decided or are considering – willingly or otherwise – to join the exodus from NYC to greener pastures" (Into the Unknown, 2022). The group's self-description reflects the urgency and anxiety related to the decision to leave the city:

> This is an inclusive group for NYC residents. We're scared. And sad. And frightened. And excited. And worried. And wondering. And hopeful. And might return. And might not, but really just have no fucking clue what is going on or what's best for us or our family.
>
> *(Into the Unknown, 2022)*

According to Rebekah Rosier, the group's founder, the experiences of those who have left the city ranges from delight with their new homes to disenchantment sparked by living in isolation and contending with fewer resources (such healthcare) as well as being overburdened by home maintenance issues companies (Lasky, 2022). As a former Soho resident who moved to Columbia County explained to me:

> I loved the peace and quiet but my wife and girls were going nuts. In the beginning, the girls loved being outside. They grew tired of it, though. They're from the city. They're used to a packed schedule with classes – acting, dance, going to the theater and museums. Country life doesn't offer that.

For Christmas 2021, I received a gift from my husband that represents the link between living in the city and one's identity. The gift was a black-and-white photograph of a historic city movie theater. The marquee read "It's New York or It's Nowhere." He shared that he found the photograph meaningful because we have been through so much in the city and that we still stand by it and love all that it has to offer. I agree. However, I am not the only person in agreement. According to a New York City Comptroller Office report (2021), based on U.S. Postal Service change-of-address forms, migration patterns for New York reversed, with more people moving back to neighborhoods that experienced the greatest flight. Therefore, the next narrative of the exodus might focus on this new stage, the return, the process of rejoining life in the city and, perhaps, a deeper appreciation of its culture and its citizenry.

Notes

1 *The New York Times* analysis drew from three studies: a Descartes Lab aggregate mobility report, a working paper by Joshua Coven and Arpit Gupta of NYU Stern School of Business, and a Teralytics report that analyzed migration patterns based on data from cellular phone patterns. All the three studies estimate New York's population change to be roughly 5% citywide with Manhattan experiencing the highest population

loss. As listed by Quealy (2020), their population change estimates for New York and Manhattan, respectively, are as follows: Descartes Labs (–5.2%; –18.6%); Coven & Gupta (–4.0%;–12.9%), and Teralytics (–5.3%; –13.7%).

2 In the 2020 U.S. Presidential election, more than 60% of Staten Island residents voted for Trump, which was an increase from the 56% of votes for Trump in 2016 (Fitzsimmons & Petri, 2020).

3 Through Instagram posts, writer/actor Jill Kargman shared a hilarious and scathing portrayal of Dzanielle, a fictional, wealthy Upper-East-Sider, who was attempting to cope with the pandemic. Kargman was lauded for using humor to call attention to how the wealthy escaped the city (Ruiz, 2020a). In each Instagram video, Dzanielle moans about having to contend with unexpected elements of her changing city; for example, dealing with tough challenges like the closing of Soul Cycle and the end of girls' lunches, she is compelled to light a Jo Malone candle to keep her sanity (My recommendation is English Pear & Freesia. Lime Basil & Mandarin is a bit too crisp for such a moment). Standing on a desolate Madison Avenue, Dzanielle complains about how it's become a ghost town and charges that some people "are cheating on New York with Hamptons." Dzanielle was right. Posh New Yorkers were so cheating on the city with the Hamptons. Their affair was shameless.

References

Bach, T. (2020, September 21). The 10 U.S. cities with the largest income gaps. *U.S. News and World Report*. www.usnews.com/news/cities/articles/2020-09-21/us-cities-with-the-biggest-income-inequality-gaps

Bachelard, G. (1958). *The poetics of space* (2nd ed., Jolas, M., Trans.). Beacon Press.

Baker, K. (2020, August 27). Affluence killed New York, not the pandemic. *The Atlantic*. www.theatlantic.com/ideas/archive/2020/08/who-new-york/615715/

Bellafante, G. (2020, March 14). The rich have a coronavirus cure: Escape from New York. *The New York Times*. www.nytimes.com/2020/03/14/nyregion/Coronavirus-nyc-rich-wealthy-residents.html

Bernstein, J. (2021a, April 15). Some New Yorkers don't want the superrich to return. *The New York Times*. www.nytimes.com/2021/04/15/style/rich-people-fled-new-york.html

Bernstein, J. (2021b, May 29). As the Hamptons boom, a new world of luxury problems. *The New York Times*. www.nytimes.com/2021/05/29/style/hamptons-summer-2021.html

Blecher, G. (2020, May 16). I left my troubled city behind. Now I feel guilty. *The New York Times*. www.nytimes.com/2020/05/16/nyregion/coronavirus-leaving-nyc.html

Brown Harris Stevens. (2021). *Year end 2020 Hamptons residential market report*. http://media.bhsusa.com/pdf/2020YearEndHamptonsMarketReport

Burton, A. (2020, March 24). Upstate counties urge New York City residents to stay in primary homes. *The New York Times*. www.wsj.com/articles/upstate-counties-urge-new-york-city-residents-to-stay-in-primary-homes-11585092090

Carey, B., & Glanz, J. (2020, May 7). Travel from New York City seeded wave of U.S. outbreaks. *The New York Times*. www.nytimes.com/2020/05/07/us/new-york-city-coronavirus-outbreak.html

Carmiel, O. (2020, October 8). Manhattan apartments haven't been this cheap to rent since 2013. *Bloomberg*. www.bloomberg.com/news/articles/2020-10-08/manhattan-apartments-haven-t-been-this-cheap-to-rent-since-2013

Clarke, K. (2020, August 20). COVID-19 pounds New York real estate worse than 9/11, financial crash. *The Wall Street Journal*. www.wsj.com/articles/covid-19-new-york-real-estate-11597939146

Coven, J., & Gupta, A. (2020, May 15). Disparities in mobility responses to COVID-19. *Squarespace*. https://static1.squarespace.com/static/56086d00e4b0fb7874bc2d42/t/5ebf201183c6f016ca3abd91/1589583893816/DemographicCovid.pdf

Douglas Elliman's Real Estate. (2021). *2020 market report*. www.elliman.com/corporate-resources/market-reports

Fitzsimmons, E., & Petri, A. (2020, November 11). How N.Y.C.'s conservative bastion became a virus hot spot. *The New York Times*. www.nytimes.com/2020/11/11/nyregion/staten-island-second-wave.html

Gould, J. (2020, March 18). Chic Hamptons food stores ransacked by the wealthy amid coronavirus pandemic. *New York Post*. https://nypost.com/2020/03/18/chic-hamptons-food-stores-ransacked-by-the-wealthy-amid-coronavirus-pandemic/

Into the Unknown. (n.d.). [About grouppage]. *Facebook*. Retrieved March 28, 2022, from www.facebook.com/groups/intotheunknownn

Lasky, J. (2022, February 25). They fled for greener pastures, and there were weeds. *The New York Times*. www.nytimes.com/2022/02/25/realestate/new-yorkers-return-nyc-pandemic.html

Mazzei, P., Bosman, J., & Bougel-Boroughs, N. (2020, March 25). Governors tell outsiders from "hot zone" to stay away as virus divides states. *The New York Times*. www.nytimes.com/2020/03/25/us/coronavirus-united-states.html

Miller, J. (2020, August 6). Why is it so hard to say goodbye to New York? *The New York Times*. www.nytimes.com/2021/08/06/realestate/leaving-new-york-city.html

New York City Comptroller. (2021, November 15). *Comptroller Stringer analysis: returningto New York Cityafter out-migrationtripled duringpandemic [Pressrelease]*. https://comptroller.nyc.gov/newsroom/comptroller-stringer-analysis-residents-returning-to-new-york-city-after-out-migration-tripled-during-pandemic/

O'Hara, J. (1934). *Appointment in Samarra*. Carpetbagger Books.

Quealy, K. (2020, May 15). The richest neighborhoods emptied out most as coronavirus hit New York City. *The New York Times*. www.nytimes.com/interactive/2020/05/15/upshot/who-left-new-york-coronavirus.html

Ruiz, M. (2020a, May 6). How Jill Kargman created Dzanielle, the quarantine comedy character we all needed. *Vogue*. www.vogue.com/article/jill-kargman-interview-dzanielle-instagram-videos

Ruiz, M. (2020b, June 17). A tale of two New Yorks: Those who left during the pandemic, and those who stayed. *Vanity Fair*. www.vanityfair.com/style/2020/06/new-yorkers-who-left-and-stayed-during-the-pandemic

Rushkoff, D. (2023). *Survival of the richest: Escape fantasies of the tech billionaires* (1st ed.). W.W. Norton & Company, Inc.

Schwartz, N. (2020). *The velvet rope economy: How inequality became big business*. Doubleday.

Skousen, J., & Skousen, A. (2011). *Strategic relocation: North American guide to safe places*. Joel Skousen Designs.

Sussman Fischler, M. (2021, May 14). The Hampton boom continues. *The New York Times*. www.nytimes.com/2021/05/14/realestate/hamptons-real-estate-sales.html

Tully, T., & Stowe, S. (2020, March 5). The wealthy flee coronavirus. Vacation towns respond: Stay away. *The New York Times*. www.nytimes.com/2020/03/25/nyregion/coronavirus-leaving-nyc-vacation-homes.html

4

SETTING UP

Prepper Closets

In the future, when Americans share their memories of the height of the COVID-19 pandemic, their discussions will center on their personal experiences and reflect on how key figures helped them to address the challenges of the pandemic (or failed to help them). Of course, everyone's memories will be unique but the key figures will most likely include elected officials such as the President, respective state and local politicians, and public health officials. These noteworthy leaders will be critiqued according to how their leadership and actions inspired a sense of hope and reassurance in people. Those memories will be valuable, but they will also be flawed. Most people will probably forget to mention a very noteworthy figure, the person who was really the first guide that helped us understand the dangers of a pandemic and how our lives would change. Matt Damon. That's right, Matt Damon.

Contagion, Steven Soderbergh's 2011 thriller that depicts the near-collapse of the world in the wake of a pandemic, became one of the top movies of 2020. As people began to fear COVID-19 and as they sought to understand what life might be like during a pandemic, the movie was streamed all over the world. At the end of 2019, *Contagion* was listed as number 270 among Warner Brother catalogue titles. At the start of 2020, *Contagion* skyrocketed to second place, bested only by a Harry Potter movie (Sperling, 2020). In the film, a virus easily transmitted through touch quickly spreads across the globe, killing 26 million people. While scientists rush to find a vaccine, a father (Matt Damon) struggles to guide his family through the perils of the pandemic as he confronts challenges ranging from the loss of his wife (patient zero) to managing food scarcity,

DOI: 10.4324/9781003400356-4

to coping with isolation. One March 2020 viewer commented on IMDb (Internet Movie Database):

> As I am watching the spread of Covid-19, I see numerous parallels with the film . . . it is describing exactly what is happening now. . . . It is therefore important to note the predictions of this film: idiots spreading rumors online, violence from desperate people, supply shortages on every level.
> *(IMDB, n.d.)*

When comparing the film to his experience living in the pandemic, one urban prepper sighed and said:

> It really is just like *Contagion*. COVID spreads so damn fast and so easily. You know, it's about trying to get your mind around it. Sure, you've got your stores and all you need. But, it's about the gradual, the ordinariness of it, the everyday bullshit, that's the real madness.

Chapters 4 and 5 of this book take on that madness by exploring NYC preppers' experiences of sheltering in place in the city – from planning for the pandemic to enduring the struggles of living through an extended period of confinement. This chapter explores prepping as a lifestyle that requires a commitment to learning and readiness. It also describes the strategies of sheltering in place such as the mastery of homesteading and first aid skills. The significance of the prepper closet as a critical tool for survival is also explored. Like many other wealthy residents of New York, high-net-worth (HNW) preppers relied on their "apocalypse insurance"[1] to escape the dangers of COVID by retreating to their hideaway destinations (Osnos, 2017, p. 39). Reflecting the split between classes in New York, HNW preppers did, in fact, split.

A pandemic is 1 of 10 scenarios for which the Federal Emergency Management Agency offers sheltering-in-place guidance.[2] Regarding pandemics, the Department of Homeland Security provides public guidance on the use of masks, good hygiene practices, physical distancing, and gathering supplies (FEMA, n.d.). For preppers, planning for disasters is a much more comprehensive process. Their preparations involve more than maintaining food and essential supplies, water storage, and sealing one's shelter against contaminants[3] if needed. As Lisa Bedford, a bestselling author of preparedness books and a popular YouTube channel creator known as "The Survival Mom" explains, prepping is a dedicated lifestyle:

> Becoming better prepared for the future isn't a single task or focus. In fact, focusing on just one element – food storage, for example – will leave your family vulnerable in other areas. Preparedness doesn't happen overnight

> or even in a month or two. Instead, it's a way of life, a new awareness of current events and trends, and a commitment to stay focused on what will help strengthen and ready your family for whatever comes along with a willingness to learn new things.
>
> *(2012, p. 28)*

Prior to the COVID-19 pandemic, NYC preppers stored provisions because they believed that New York's food network could be disrupted in the event of a disaster. Hunts Point, located in the Bronx, is the city's largest food distribution facility as it supplies produce and meat to nearly half of the city's restaurants. Sections of the 60-acre facility, such as its meat market, are in low-lying areas and may be prone to flooding during heavy storms, while other sections on higher ground might be subject to power outages (Hester, 2017). Concerns about the scarcity of food during disaster also influenced preppers to learn food preservation techniques. In addition to buying local foods and attempting to grow some items, preppers practice canning, freezing, and drying methods to store food.

Audrey, an Asian-American NYC prepper who learned about planning for disaster while growing up in Hawaii (which is prone to hurricanes and fires caused by periodic volcano eruptions), agrees that prepping is a lifestyle choice that permeates all decision-making and aspects of life. Prepping for her is not merely a response to protect one's family from a specific disaster like the pandemic. To clarify her point, she shared her experience of shopping for a home in the city. According to Audrey, her approach to reviewing potential homes was much more complex because it involved a deeper investigation into issues like building safety and neighborhood safety. As she explained:

> My move from Soho to the Bronx is a great example that prepping is a perspective that influences everything. For me, when it came to building safety, I wasn't just interested in the building. I wanted to know about the ground that it was build it on. How safe was it? The apartment building was constructed on bedrock. It is a strong foundation that will hold up. Also, most people don't really do a thorough safety check of the neighborhood. They just look at surface things. I wanted to be sure that I knew what my new neighborhood would be like 24–7. I walked around at night to see what stores were open 24 hours, where I could go to if someone was following me, like a deli or drugstore. Also, I wanted to know about which buildings had entrances open at night that I could slip into if needed. These things matter. Most people don't consider them.

Inshirah, a former Brooklyn prepper who now lives in New Jersey, holds a similar perspective about preparedness as a lifestyle. For her, being a prepper requires a tremendous ongoing commitment to increasing one's knowledge and to developing skills. When asked if having a store of provisions meant that people were engaging in prepping, her response was swift:

> No, that doesn't make you a prepper. Let's say you are a person with a lot of canned food with a can opener. What if you lose or break your can opener? Well, then you are just a regular person with a lot of cans.

While humorous, Inshirah's response reinforces the prepper's adage of: "Two is one, one is none." A prepper would have a tested back-up plan and probably two for obtaining food rather than relying solely on the use of one tool.

For preppers, the goal of sheltering in place is to protect your family by creating an organized, well-stocked, and safe refuge from the dangers of the outside world. Central to the success of this mission is being prepared in advance by the creation of a "prepper closet." A prepper closet is a designated storage area that contains critical supplies for use during emergencies. For New Yorkers who must adapt to smaller dwellings, a prepper closet is not always a closet. My research in New York confirms that any dedicated space can be transformed into a prepper closet including a cabinet, the floor underneath a bed, as well as furniture with hidden storage like ottomans and couches. Prepper closets are also viewed as a viable strategy for preparing against disaster because home ownership is not required. Renters can easily create a prepper closet without permission from their landlords.

Typically, prepper closets contain items from a common set of categories: nonperishable food, medical supplies (including masks and hand sanitizer), water (containers, water bobs), light sources (such as headlamps, flashlights, and lanterns), power sources (batteries, solar-charging pads), tools and supplies for sealing off a home against contaminants (duct tape, plastic lining, tarp). While they do hold similar items, each prepper closet is carefully curated to satisfy the preferences and needs of their particular household. Beyond first aid kits, medical supplies may also include prescription medications and extra contact lens or glasses. Protective gear like masks (surgical and gas), disposable gloves, and the occasional Hazmat suit are also cached. Food provisions may include not just freeze-dried meals but homemade goods like tomato sauce and preserved fruits. Snack possibilities can range from nut and granola bars to expensive chocolate. Alcoholic beverages and liquor are also sometimes stored.[4] Special rewards like coloring books, young adult fiction, and games are also stored to entertain bored children and to boost their spirits. According to experienced preppers, food should not be selected just because it has a long storage life. Instead, it should be chosen for being relatively healthful and something that the family typically consumes. For example, Jason encourages people to store freeze-dried foods or select canned goods that have a high nutritional value. Marlon, the leader of the UOS, explains, "There is no need for you to buy a tub of disgusting goo because someone is trying to sell it to you. You should be storing things that your family will enjoy eating."

Just as Jason's influence in the prepping world is enormous, so, too, is his prepper closet, a reflection of his commitment to preparedness and his curiosity about testing prepping gear. Consisting of one apartment closet and a 100-square-foot storage unit, his prepper closet is intended to help his family survive in any type of disaster. With stores of canned foods found on sale, freeze-dried meals, vats of pasta and rice, as well as MREs (Meals Ready to Eat), Jason has enough food to feed his family for a year. During meetings, he has occasionally offered a humorous taste test report on expired foods when rotating out outdated goods. His prepping gear is extensive, ranging from an inflatable raft to be used on the Hudson River, and a cache of 100 knives, to drones for determining which areas of the neighborhood are safe.

While preppers do not often reveal the contents of their prepper closets to avoid stigma and to protect their provisions, Jason's interest in educating people about preparedness has outweighed this precaution. To a non-prepper, Jason's prepper closet might be viewed as an example of hoarding or as evidence of membership in a fringe survivalist group. However, as a prepping group leader, he often tests and demonstrates the use of equipment. For example, a recent Instagram post shows his collection of bugout bags that he has used throughout the years. Jason's knife collection also stems from his interest in knife collecting and receiving knives as promotional items rather than amassing weapons for Armageddon. While non-preppers view knives only as weapons, preppers recognize the value of knives in survival tasks such as building a shelter, crafting tools, and hunting. Based on his interest in bushcraft and survival skills, Jason tests knives and shares his reviews on his social media websites and among preppers. He also teaches knife skills workshops at group events (and displays different types of knives for review). For preppers, Jason is demonstrating his knowledge and skill by testing products and educating others about their proper use. Jason's prepper closet extends beyond storing provisions to also function as a teacher's supply cabinet.

Given its importance in a crisis, a prepper closet is considered "off-limits" to the family in ordinary situations. This strategy prevents borrowing from the closet, ensuring that it remains stocked with needed supplies for use during emergencies. Unlike most New Yorkers, NYC preppers interviewed for my research had already developed plans for protecting their families against the spread of a deadly virus. Weeks before the virus hit New York, NYC preppers were double-checking their stores and securing their information and resource networks. Prior to the pandemic, Audrey's prepper closet already held many items that would be useful (and hard to find) during the outbreak. She had already stockpiled a few N-95 masks, an ozone generator to sanitize rooms, nitrile gloves, hydrogen peroxide, and white vinegar for additional sanitizing, and some Tyvek (protective) clothing. In preparing for a possible outbreak, Audrey purchased additional protective gear: "I ordered more PPE [Personal Protective Equipment] for myself and for my parents. I also ordered more vitamins and supplements mostly for respiratory support. I didn't trust that what was going around was just SARS COV-2." Her food stores included canned mackerel and sardines, canned chili and corned beef hash, Kim Chee and sauerkraut, 15-pound bags of white rice, brussel sprouts, potatoes and shallots (which have longer shelf lives than other vegetables. She also had 90 lbs. of mung beans for sprouting which she and her son could live on for a year if necessary. Again, personal preferences are important. Audrey also explained that she began collecting SPAM late in the lockdown: "I hoarded SPAM. Bacon Spam is the best." I agree. Since SPAM was first introduced in 1937, there are now 10 different varieties of this pork product. Over 9 billion cans have been sold with Hawaii consuming over seven million cans every year (Hormel Foods, n.d.).

In late January 2020, I received a call from Ron, one of the urban preppers with whom I'd spent a lot of time on excursions while writing my first book. We had been through quite a lot together in the field. Well, I had been through a lot and Ron was an excellent mentor. He rescued my tent when it had the nerve to blow away. Ron also kept me from freezing to death on an overnight excursion to the beach. We have maintained contact, periodically sharing our perspectives on topics like the news, prepping strategies, and ghost sightings by our older relatives. Our calls are usually light-hearted and entertaining. I always learn something. During this call, I learned how concerned he was about the possibility of a national shelter-in-place order. He wanted to go over my preps with me, specifically the type of provisions and the number of days that I was planning for, to be sure that I would be ready to stay in. He ran over a checklist with me. I passed his test, but I had just 2 weeks of provisions. His advice was to acquire a full month's supply. He also shared that I could reach out to him if I needed specific supplies, as he had contacts. I could hear the concern in his voice. We both sensed that trouble was ahead.

A few weeks later, a colleague sent a funny photo of people panic shopping for toilet paper at a big box store in New Jersey. He asked, "Know any of these preppers from your research?" His question reminded me of the misunderstanding that people have about preppers. Panic buying at inflated prices is exactly what preppers plan *not* to do. As COVID-19 made staying at home a necessity for many Americans in 2020, they adopted basic prepping practices such as securing food and essential items to provide for their families. However, as Ron pointed out to me weeks later, trying to survive the pandemic does not make you a prepper. Rather, prepping requires an ongoing commitment. He explained:

> Right now, people are definitely trying to prepare and look out for their families. What we do is different, though. It's hard to prepare for all things.

> First, it takes time to figure out what you need and the skills you need to learn. Then, it takes time to learn new skills and to get up your supplies. We pay attention to things. We talk and exchange information ahead of regular people.

In contrast to buying survival items only in response to the threat of COVID-19, NYC preppers already had prepper closets, stockpiles of food and supplies in their apartments to help their families during a sheltering-in-place emergency. Unlike the precarious stacks of toilet paper, cases of Kombucha bottles and jars of spaghetti sauce that were jammed in the living rooms or bedrooms of many New Yorkers,[5] the emergency stores of urban preppers were well-organized units that reflected tremendous investments of labor, time, and money. Given the urgent deadline to gather supplies for staying at home, many Americans tried to quickly figure out what to buy by watching news reports as well as checking out prepper websites and YouTube videos. Most Americans bought food supplies at places like big box stores and grocery stores, both in-person and online. During the shopping frenzy, a second friend texted a photo of another packed big box store with customers actually fighting with one another over toilet paper. She commented that "the preppers were out in full force and ready to throw down." She was wrong. The crazed shoppers weren't preppers. The preppers were at home. They were already set. The shoppers were scared and panicked people.

It is worth noting that Americans reacted quite differently in response to the Avian Flu in 2006. At that time, George W. Bush's Secretary of Health and Human Services (HHS), Mike Leavitt urged Americans to stock up on canned goods and provisions as preparation for a possible Avian Flu pandemic (Moena, 2006). The Secretary of HHS was perceived as an alarmist and ridiculed in the popular media. On the Tonight Show, host Jay Leno quipped, "Secretary of Health and Human Services Michael Leavitt recommended that Americans store canned tuna and powdered milk under their beds for when bird flu hits. "What? . . . Powdered milk and tuna? How many would rather have the bird flu?" (Diamond, 2020). Later, Secretary Leavitt described the Catch-22 experienced by health and national security officials in trying to get alert the public: Prepare too early and you're called Chicken Little. Act too late – and millions may die. In advance of a pandemic, anything you say sounds alarmist. After a pandemic starts, everything you've done is inadequate" (Diamond, 2020).

Unlike the shopping experience depicted in the photo, selecting and storing food supplies for one's closet is a painstaking and complex process for preppers. Many Americans panic-shopped at grocery stores just before the pandemic and often paid higher prices. According to the U.S Department of Agriculture (Chelius & MacLachlan, 2021), grocery store food prices increased by 3.5% on average from 2019 to 2020 (75% higher than the

20-year historical level of retail food price inflation of 2% a year). Furthermore, prices for every major food-at-home category increased in 2020 with the exception of fresh fruits.[6] Moreover, by slowly stocking up during normal circumstances, preppers were able to better plan purchases. Preppers had time to research products before buying them. Preppers could also wait to buy items on sale or take the time to find inexpensive substitutes for costly items. Given their interest in self-reliance and their concerns about financial disaster – whether global or personal – careful spending and saving money are important goals for preppers. For many urban preppers, the need to prepare for lean times has also been learned from family traditions and growing up in immigrant communities. Isabella, a Brooklyn prepper who was raised in a large Mexican family, explains:

> My dad worked construction and my mom was a homemaker. Every week, she planned our dinners around what was in the sale ads. Amazing cook. She could transform anything into a good meal. Warm homemade tortillas always filled us up. She would add corn to hamburger to make the dish bigger. She treated a trip to the dollar store like a treasure hunt – no junk, only worthwhile things. She'd buy spices and all sorts of canned food. I try to do the same now.

For preppers, careful planning for stores of food also involves repackaging dry goods to extend their shelf life or to expand the number of servings. (Many dry goods such as rice or pasta come in packing that is not durable. The food may become stale quickly or become infested with insects.) During the first stage of the pandemic, Isabella gave me a tour of her prepper closet via Facetime. In her late thirties, Isabella wore her dark hair up in a bun. She was bare-faced and dressed in a close-fitting athletic shirt and yoga pants. (Later, we would all be wearing this same pandemic outfit.) She stored her emergency provisions in an oversized Ikea wardrobe with sliding doors. Stationed in her bedroom, it looked like it was being used to store clothes rather than supplies to survive a disaster. However, after she slid a door open, I could see that Isabella and her husband had "DIYed" the wardrobe by adding shelving of various heights after having removed the clothes rod.[7] Instead of being used to store long items like bulky coats, long dresses, and suits, their wardrobe housed an organized collection of labeled glass and plastic containers as well as canned foods. Their provisions fell into three main categories: food, medical, and tools. Isabella's prepper closet reflected the careful approach of preppers in shopping and storing food. All dry goods like flour or pasta that were originally packed in paper bags or paper boxes had been transferred into glass containers to extend their shelf life. Isabella explained that paper packaging could easily tear or become damp. Worse yet, it could also be subject to infestation by rodents or insects. Organized by type of meal, groups of freeze-dried meals, both homemade and store-bought, were placed in plastic containers. The serving sizes of some of the store-bought camping meals had been expanded by adding more rice. Canned foods included both home-canned items like tomatoes and peaches, and store-bought cans of meats such as tuna, mackerel, and salmon, as well as vegetables. Nontoxic oxygen absorbers were also packed with some foods like rice, beans, and oatmeal. Given the continued coverage of toilet paper shortages in the media, I asked her about how she stored extra toilet paper in an apartment. She pulled out a plastic tub and took off the lid to reveal about two dozen flattened rolls of toilet paper. The cardboard inner rolls had actually been removed to save space.

Among preppers, Isabella's interest in canning and making preserves is not unusual. Many preppers practice homesteading skills such as gardening, canning, and drying foods. Prepping in the city is rooted in the philosophy of urban homesteading, which involves striving for self-sufficiency and practicing sustainable living strategies. Popular urban homesteading activities include growing produce or buying locally produced food, home canning and preserving, bee keeping, and raising chickens, as well as restoring and upcycling goods (re-purposing items for alternative uses). To supply their prepper closets, New York preppers rely on growing their own produce, shopping at green markets, and ordering provisions directly from farmers. Given that most apartments lack outdoor space, some NYC preppers grow produce in compact indoor garden systems, in traditional container gardens, or in window boxes. Herbs, fruits, vegetables, and greens are grown for consumption and preservation. Given advancements in lighting, growing techniques, and even in the design of plant containers, the possibilities of indoor gardening have proliferated. Isabella had a compact Aero Garden unit with a grow light on her kitchen counter, filled with herbs such as basil, dill, and oregano. She has also used it to grow cherry tomatoes. Renee, a prepper in Manhattan, has a large, hydroponic garden tower in her oversized living room. The beautiful, white, round unit looked more like sculpture with its little bouquets of lettuce bursting out of their pockets.[8]

In addition to gardening at home, some preppers grow vegetables and herbs in community gardens. New York's collection of community gardens, known as GreenThumb, is the nation's largest gardening program with 550 gardens and thousands of volunteer gardeners throughout the city (NYC Parks, n.d.). Beyond community gardens, preppers also rely on New York's growing network of communal and commercial farms. Preppers sometimes subscribe to food-box programs (boxes delivered from farmers). These subscription services enable customers to minimize contact by picking up food at a designated location (with fewer people than grocery stores) or by having deliveries placed outside their doors. Communal farms are operated by nonprofits that serve the nearby communities through food production and programming (information sessions and events); commercial farms focus on maximizing profitability while also helping to shape urban agricultural goals (Bauer & Fletcher, 2014). Both types of farming include a mix of traditional farms, vertical indoor farms, and rooftop farms. A recent surprising example of a New York City farm is the 8-acre rooftop farm that sits atop the Javits Center. The rooftop farm was created through a partnership between NYC Audubon and Brooklyn Grange, a green roof company. In addition to serving as a bird sanctuary amid concrete and asphalt, the Javits Farm grows at least 16,000 pounds of produce per year (Misdary, 2023).

NYC preppers also shop at greenmarkets throughout the city for fresh produce to can or dry. New York has the largest open air greenmarket program in the country. New York has 50 greenmarkets that support 240 farmers throughout the region (GrowNYC, 2018). Larger greenmarkets such as the Union Square Greenmarket also offer various plant-based goods like essential oils or tonics. Given their long shelf life, these alternative medicines are often stored by preppers. Examples of products available include essential oils like Lavender (to soothe aching muscles) and Elderberry cough medicine.

To develop their homesteading skills, these preppers attend classes or events related to the topics of gardening, canning, or preserving food. Preppers who belong to organized groups then demonstrate and teach their skills at meetings. Preppers also attend classes and other types of training outside of the group. Challenging wilderness survival courses are quite popular. Audrey has even taken an online fishing class offered by the Boy Scouts which she thought was terrific. Preppers also exchange information informally through conversations, exchanging details about various experiences and methods. For example, before the pandemic, the NYCPN periodically conducted demonstrations or held hands-on workshops so that members could learn how to preserve food through canning or drying. In keeping with the prepping philosophy of self-reliance, the workshops were useful because members were provided not just with instruction but with the opportunity to work with tools and equipment. However, these skills demand commitment, as achieving mastery often requires additional practice beyond the group workshops.

After attending a homesteading workshop on making fruit preserves one fall, I left with a tiny jar of strawberry jam. I felt like a pioneer woman. The next weekend, I experienced delight in spreading the jam over some toast. It was delicious. I was heady and empowered. I just knew that I could save my family from starvation through my new-found expertise in fruit preservation. Finally, I could leave behind me that grade of "D" I received in Home Economics. Pretending to be Aunt Bee on some ancient episode of *The Andy Griffith Show*, I decided that I would make and give homemade jam as Christmas gifts for my extended family members. Everyone received scented candles that year. I had wasted a million dollars on strawberries. I exploded some jars. Sometimes, a thin, white, stringy layer would appear over the jam in surviving jars (Yes, just like in *The Last of Us*.) I did not perfect my jam technique until well after Valentine's Day. I did not discuss this experience with Isabella.

Water is also essential. The general recommendation is to have two gallons of water stored per person, per day. Meeting this guideline is challenging for apartment dwellers as storing water takes up a tremendous amount of space. Therefore, NYC preppers rely on several water storage strategies. For example, in addition to the extra water that she stored in her kitchen, Isabella had six, one-gallon water containers stored on the bottom shelf of her closet. Like many other preppers, Isabella planned to fill her bathtub with water if needed. For this, she kept on hand a WaterBOB, a tub liner designed to protect water from soap and film. She also stored a bottle of unscented bleach to treat contaminated water.[9] A bathtub usually holds about 100 gallons of water. If using the bathtub water for drinking only, Isabella and her husband would have water for 25 days.

Medical supplies are the second category of emergency stores. In preparation for the pandemic, many Americans bought extra supplies of over-the-counter medicines like Tylenol or Benadryl as well as refills of prescription medication. And, of course, there was a mad dash for hand sanitizer. In 2020, U.S. sales of hand sanitizers increased by 600%, totaling roughly $1.3 billion in sales (Terlep, 2021). For Isabella, medical supplies ranged from over-the-counter medicines to treat common ailments like pain or allergies to prescription drugs as well as extra contact lens and glasses for both Isabella and her husband to an advanced first aid kit for wounds and burns. Her prepper closet also contained a collection of essential oils and several boxes of surgical masks and gloves as well as large bottles of hand sanitizer. Again, reflecting greater preparation for disasters, Isabella had taken first aid training to improve her knowledge of wound care. Isabella explained:

> My husband and I had gone over our bugging-in scenarios. We knew that we would need to treat whatever we could at home because there might not be access to a hospital. Now, we know that we want to stay away from the emergency room. I have some training but we also have books and YouTube if we can't reach someone – not ideal, but safer than ER.

During the first 3 months of the pandemic, New York City hospitals were often overwhelmed by seriously ill coronavirus patients and those with infectious diseases and pneumonia; however, there was a significant drop in the number of patients who typically come to the emergency room for care (Abelson, 2020).

Like Isabella, many NYC preppers receive training to provide medical care to better protect their families during dire circumstances when these services may not be available. Courses like the Red Cross's First Aid Certification and

First Aid for Severe Trauma (how to control bleeding) are popular among preppers. Advanced courses like Wilderness First Aid are also often taken because they provide instruction on how to treat injuries that occur in the outdoors like fractures and head injuries until qualified help arrives.

In their bestselling reference book for preppers, *The Survival Medicine Handbook: The Essential Guide for When Help is Not on the Way*, Alton and Alton (2021) acknowledge the challenges of planning to provide medical care in a survival situation. Emergency medicine is based on the practice of temporary care to "stabilize and transport" until the person reaches a medical facility; however, in a disaster, there may be no access to medical care. As Alton and Alton (2021, p. 11) note, during a disaster, "You go from being a temporary first-aid provider to being the caregiver at the end of the line . . . the highest medical resource." While these authors argue that increased knowledge and training for nonphysicians is valuable, they acknowledge that these measures cannot replace modern medical care and equipment for severe issues. Still, they argue that preppers need to be ready for "the long haul" (Alton & Alton, 2021; p. 11). In preparation for a lengthy period without access to medical care or during a medication shortage, some preppers store alternative therapies or substitute medicines for prescription drugs that may be unavailable. Essential oils are often used to treat common ailments such as stomach aches or muscle soreness. In addition, certain oils are considered to be useful in helping to stop bleeding. Fearful that they may not have access to important antibiotics, some preppers store substitutes. For example, some preppers believe fish antibiotics to be viable substitutes for antibiotics designed for humans. When I first learned of this strategy, I didn't understand. I kept thinking that the prepper was referring to some type of over-the-counter pills that contain fish ingredients such as Omega-5 fish oil pills often recommended for the heart. No, this knowledgeable and highly skilled prepper was referring to the flecks that you sprinkle into a tank to help your fish when it has an infection – an over-the-counter product readily available at pet stores. I have learned all sorts of skills and tips from urban preppers – from making fire to building a shelter to treating open chest wounds. Eating fish medicine? I was skeptical and, well, a little freaked out. Without question, it seemed wildly risky.

Also, I have a bias. I have never believed that fish medicine even works for fish. After all, I'd lost Ricky. In the second grade, I came home from school one day to discover that my sweet goldfish, Ricky, had passed in spite of our efforts to cure his infection. His bowl was on my dresser. I always fed him right after school. With tears streaming, I ran to my mother who was in the kitchen. After hearing the heartbreaking news, she turned off the stove and affirmed her love for Ricky too. She told me to have a seat on the couch while she made preparations for the service. I took a seat. A few minutes later, my mother marched through the living room to my bedroom with a few tools, a big metal spoon, and a small plastic soup container from our favorite Chinese take-out place. She told me to meet her in the backyard. Walking very solemnly, my mom carried out Ricky in the little soup container. She had the big spoon under her arm. She chose a spot in the back corner of the yard as the grave site. While she dug the tiny grave with her spoon, I pretended to look for dandelions but kept eyeballing my mom's gorgeous yellow tulips until she relented. After burying Ricky, now free from the burdens of this world, including the soup container, my mom and I held hands as she said a short prayer and wished him happiness in the heavenly oceans. I sang a few bars of *He's Got the Whole World in His Hands*.

Leaving my thoughts of Ricky aside, I continued to investigate the use of fish antibiotics as a substitute for antibiotics made for humans. According to the prepper, the antibiotics are relatively the same and the challenge is being sure that you use the correct dosage. While I am by no means recommending the substitution of animal antibiotics for human antibiotics, this strategy does reflect the level of planning and the inventiveness of preppers in seeking to save lives in emergency situations. Is this an effective and safe treatment in an emergency situation? The answer, with several cautionary caveats, is a strong "maybe." First, there is the challenge of a layperson determining the correct antibiotic to treat a specific infection without medical testing. Next, calculating the correct dosage when the antibiotics are in varying forms – for example, a pill versus powder – would be extremely difficult. Furthermore, there is the question of human-grade antibiotics that are in time-released pill form. However, the majority of fish antibiotics are identical to human antibiotics in both dosages and form such as color, shape, pills, or capsule.[10] Still, the consumption or absence of excipient ingredients could also be very dangerous. For example, many human-grade antibiotics in pill form have a special coating to prevent damage to the stomach lining which may not be present in fish antibiotics. Popescu-Roberts et al. (2022) found that both prescribed, human-grade and over-the-counter commercially available fish forms of the antimicrobials amoxicillin and cephalexin met required standards and are pharmacologically indistinguishable. While no major impurities were identified, there was evidence of several as-yet unidentified excipient ingredients. Excipient ingredients could refer to coating and dyes that may be harmless to fish but dangerous for human consumption. The consumption of fish antibiotics by humans may also reveal a severe or fatal drug allergy. Therefore, such substitutions come at high risk. However, as one registered nurse explained to me, "If you are in an apocalyptical situation without any human antibiotics and you may die from infection, you may as well take the fish flakes."

When faced with everyday disasters such as being faced with the ongoing challenges of having little money and/or no health insurance, those interested in surviving may have already made the switch. While no data is available on the number of fish antibiotics sold to consumers or on the number of those antibiotics taken by humans, the proliferation of online pet medicine suppliers and the increased support of self-diagnosing on social media and internet forums suggest that the rate of nonprescribed drug use has increased (Zhang et al., 2021; Egelund & Casapao, 2020). Furthermore, the practices of self-diagnosing, using fish antibiotics, and incorrectly dosing may also be contributing to the rise in antibiotic resistance (Egelund & Casapao, 2020).

Prepper closets are also used to store gear and tools that would be useful during a disaster. To help offset the loss of power, preppers usually stockpile items such as flashlights, extra batteries, LED lanterns, and solar-powered light disks. To receive information and to communicate, preppers also store transistor or hand-cranked radios as well as foldable solar panels designed to recharge cell phones. In addition to many of these items, Isabella kept a portable mini power generator to operate small appliances like a hot plate or to charge her laptop. She referred to it as "a giant battery."

In planning for a possible pandemic, preppers also store an array of protective equipment such as N-95 masks, face shields, disposable gloves, disinfectants, hand sanitizer, and even hazmat suits. Isabella had plenty of these items with the exception of hazmat suits. Beyond wearing protective equipment, urban preppers also set up decontamination stations near their front doors to disinfect incoming packages (mail, newspapers, and deliveries) and to remove clothing and footwear that has been worn outside. For example, Isabella shared that she always wore the same outfit whenever she left her apartment building: a long-sleeved shirt covered by a windbreaker, cargo pants (with plenty of pockets to hold her ID, credit cards, smart phone, a small bottle of sanitizer spray, and extra gloves), closed-toed shoes without laces, an N-95 mask, and a face shield, with her hair in a tidy ponytail. Once back in her apartment, she would immediately disrobe and place her dirty outfit in a new plastic bag to be placed outside the apartment door, ready to be taken to the laundry room for washing.

Given their concerns about the possibility that a lengthy shutdown might cause food shortages, some urban preppers purchased compact deep freezers to store frozen meat and other food items. The concern about possible food shortages drove some preppers to make sure that they had another piece of equipment – a weapon to protect their families. Due to NYC restrictions on firearms and knives, these preppers are often reluctant to discuss their planned self-defense strategies. Weapons seemed to range from knives, baseball bats stationed by the door to firearms. Isabella explained to me that she and her husband were very close with the other tenants in her small building and that they looked out for one another. Isabella's neighbors knew that she and her husband were interested in prepping but she said that the couple was "low key" in discussing the real level of their commitment to self-reliance. In addition to being concerned about the stigma associated with being a prepper, she also believed that "people come into prepping after they have experienced the dangers of being unprepared." Isabella became interested in preparing after Hurricane Sandy (2012). In her early twenties and living with two roommates, she realized quickly that the days without power and water would have been easier with even a few supplies. Soon after the hurricane, she began reading prepper websites and putting together a list of items that she might need in case of an emergency.

The prepper awakening (Barker, 2022) of Isabella's partner, Lucas, an African American, stems more from the resiliency that he learned as a child growing up in rural Virginia. Although his father worked full time in a factory, his family still sometimes faced the challenges of lean times. However, Lucas's lessons in resiliency did not come from learning how his parents coped with financial difficulties. Instead, he learned resilience from his father's belief in self-reliance and homesteading. His father had little faith in the dollar. You could lose your job. You might not be paid. Economic collapse could undermine its value. Therefore, his father preferred to barter for goods and services with other workers. To reduce reliance (and spending) at the grocery store, Lucas's father maintained a large garden in which they harvested fruits and vegetables ranging from plums to collards. Of course, much of the produce was preserved and put away for the winter. His father also hunted. Deer and other local game were their family's mainstay. His mother always made fresh bread. Every Sunday, the family would enjoy a large dinner. The remaining food would be stretched and supplemented with different side dishes throughout the week. According to Lucas, his childhood experiences taught him that "resiliency means not just working hard for your family's success but it's the responsibility of planning and providing for your family regardless of financial circumstances." For Lucas, being prepared for disaster is an extension of this lesson. Laughing, he also shared two more lessons from childhood: (1) He refuses to eat leftovers, and (2) He ate bear once and that was enough for a lifetime. I warned him that a pandemic was probably going to involve eating leftovers. (Isabella reports that it did.)

Based on Ron's urging and my conversations with NYC preppers like Isabella, my husband and I increased our provisions. We even bought a compact freezer. I had most of the provisions that other preppers had. I even sent ordered items online for my parents in another state to be sure that they were well-stocked. I guess you could say that I was ready. But I really wasn't. While I followed the advice of preppers in trying to protect myself and my family from the pandemic, I didn't share their same mindset. Through adopting a lifestyle of preparedness and self-reliance, they really had braced themselves for the apocalypse. My wilderness excursions with the members of the NY-CPN had toughened me up a bit. However, I had gained enough knowledge to know that I really didn't know anything.

Like so many other people, I was really worried about my family. In my first book, I wrote about my niece and my fears about being unable to secure her diabetes medication. However, the timing of the pandemic brought an unexpected fear. My niece, in her mid-twenties, was pregnant and due to give birth in October 2020. In the weeks before the pandemic, my family was overjoyed with the news. However, we all understood that her high-risk pregnancy meant trips to emergency rooms and overnight hospital stays in dangerous and overcrowded circumstances. Given the high rate of COVID infection among senior citizens, I was also worried about my older parents. Even in his late seventies, my father maintained his independent streak. He was no stranger to risk. I worried because he was widowed and lived alone. My mother, divorced from my father, also remained fiercely independent. Polite but noncompliant was her approach. I sent some provisions despite their protests. Later, when the stores were out of essentials like toilet paper and paper towels, they were grateful. Well, not really. My dad maintained that the "pandemic was blown out of proportion" for several weeks. However, he called me one day to explain that he had seen "a beautiful blonde talking about preparedness" on TV and that she had convinced him to get onboard and take it seriously. I was flattered by father's comment as I assumed that he had seen me on television. I was incorrect. It seems that my father had fallen in love with Kate Hudson on *The Ellen Show*. So much for my research.

While my husband and I prepared to shelter in place, I kept thinking about Inshirah's comments about the meaninglessness of provisions without skill. I really wasn't worried about an extra can opener. My Mexican grandmother taught me how to open a can with a big knife when I was a kid. She had a million can openers in her drawer. However, she grew up in poverty so she was used to opening them with a knife. My concern was about the loss of my reading glasses. I had three pairs stationed around the apartment – in the office, the bedroom, the living room. Still, I was worried that I would lose all three in my small Manhattan apartment. I imagined myself being trapped in my apartment with no distractions, surrounded by piles of incredible books but without my glasses. Unable to read, I would be consumed with rage and despair. Like *The Twilight Zone*'s Henry Bemis, the book lover who, after an atomic blast, finds himself alone with a library's contents of books and no glasses, I would shout, "There was *time* now; all that I needed, that's not fair!" (Season 1, Episode 8). I ordered some cheap readers just in case.

In mid-February 2020, I received a call from my favorite cousin in Texas that made me realize my level of fear. He was calling to talk over my plans to stay in the city. He does not call himself a prepper, but he shares many of the same habits of self-reliance. Since he lives in rural Texas, he makes sure that his family is prepared for disaster and that they have ample food and supplies in the event that they must stay at home for an extensive period. As kids, we faced all sorts of fears together – terrifying roller coasters, risky waterpark rides (poorly constructed and soon-to-be dismantled), and sometimes shitty parenting. As adults, we also faced our fears about the declining health of our respective fathers. My cousin asked me thoughtful questions about my provisions: "Never mind about water filtration, do you have enough Lactaid? That's the stuff that matters right now. What about that fancy tea of yours? You lose your cool when you don't have that." Yes, I had plenty of both. He asked me if I was sure that I wasn't going to leave New York. I was sure. He told me he already suspected that and he disagreed with my decision. Silent, we let the fear settle over us for a moment.

Finally, he spoke. "I have been thinking it over. We can meet halfway. I'll bring what you need in my trunk. You put the bag in your trunk and you drive back. It could be chaos there. You just don't know. You need to be ready."

My cousin rarely leaves Texas. His was an extraordinary gesture. I kept thinking about the word "ready." What does that really mean? We had no idea what was going to happen. Really, how could we be ready? For me, did being "ready" mean having guns to protect my family, if needed?

My fear did make me pause for a moment. Having grown up in the South with relatives and friends who hunt, I am not anti-gun but I support increased gun safety measures and regulation. However, my mind turned to horrific moments – not imaginary scenarios of intruders breaking into our apartment but memories of when a gun in the home has proven dangerous, like when my father pointed a .357 gun at me because he mistook me for a burglar trying to get in through the patio door – it was a surprise visit – or when I heard the news that a relative had taken his life with a gun. My fear of the known outweighed my fear of the unknown. (Schimmenti et al., 2020).

I thanked my cousin but I declined.

"I appreciate your offer and I completely understand. But I'm betting on the city. We're going to be fine."

He sighed and ended the call, "Anna, I just hope that you are right."

Notes

1 "Apocalypse Insurance" refers to how some of the extremely wealthy plan for the apocalypse from a risk management perspective.
2 The 11 scenarios are: Active Shooter, Chemical Hazard, Earthquake, Hurricane, Flooding, Nuclear Detonation, Tornado, Winter Storm, Pandemic, Thunderstorm
3 Contaminants can refer to chemical, biological, or radiological hazards. A recent example involved sealing one's windows to prevent the inhalation of smoke and ash from the Canadian Wildfires.
4 Note that sales for canned cocktails spike during March 2020. In compared to sales in March 2019, sales for Cutwater Spirits increased by 70%; Tip Top Proper cocktails rose by 50%, and Ramona (a canned wine spritzer) sales spiked by 232% (Simonson, 2020).
5 Yes, Kombucha is still a thing.

6 According to Chelius and MacLachlan (2021), the USDA reports that, in 2020, fresh fruit prices dropped by 0.8% from 2019 because of domestic and international shifts in supply and demand. International supply chain issues such as port delays and staffing shortages decreased the importation of fruit to the United States. Within the United States, the market for fruit shifted from foodservice businesses (restaurants and caterers) to retailers which also reduced prices.
7 Hacking Ikea furniture is a popular activity for DIYers and creatives, but it is also a valuable practice for preppers who wish to upcycle furniture as a homesteading practice or to modify furniture for sheltering-in-place purposes.
8 *Bracing for the Apocalypse* contains a discussion of Renee's prepper closet. Renee and her family left for their second home. Renee declined to be interviewed about her decision to leave the city and to discuss their COVID-19 experience.
9 Guidelines for disinfecting water with bleach depend on the percentage of sodium hypochlorite. Bleach typically contains 6% or 8.25% sodium hypochlorite. For Emergency Disinfection of Drinking Water instructions, see www.epa.gov/ground-water-and-drinking-water/emergency-disinfection-drinking-water.
10 Egelund and Casapao (2020) contain both information on the chemical analysis of the antibiotics as well as photo comparisons.

References

Abelson, R. (2020, June 3). E.R. visits drop sharply during pandemic. *The New York Times*. www.nytimes.com/2020/06/03/health/hospitals-coronavirus.html

Alton, J., & Alton, A. (2021). *The survival medicine handbook: The essential guide for when help is not on the way*. Doom and Bloom Medical.

Barker, K. (2022). Awakening from the sleep-walking society: Crisis, detachment and the real in prepper awakening narratives. *Environment and Planning D: Society and Space*, *40*(5), 805–823.

Bauer, C., & Fletcher, R. (Eds.). (2014). *Five borough farm phase II: Growing the benefits of urban agriculture in New York City*. Vanguard Direct.

Bedford, L. (2012). *Survival mom*. Harper One.

Chelius, C., & MacLachlan, M. (2021, March 1). Retail food price inflation in 2020 outpaced historical average by 75 %. *USDA Economic Research Servicefzhang*. www.ers.usda.gov/amber-waves/2021/march/retail-food-price-inflation-in-2020-outpaced-historical-average-by-75-%/

Diamond, D. (2020, April 11). Inside America's 2-decade failure to prepare for coronavirus. *POLITICO*. www.politico.com/news/magazine/2020/04/11/america-two-decade-failure-prepare-coronavirus-179574#:~:text=Top%20officials%20from%20three%20administrations,and%20budgets%20funded%20and%20defunded

Egelund, E. F., & Casapao, A. M. (2020). "Pet Nemo's pills": The last loophole in antimicrobial stewardship? *Clinical Infectious Diseases*, *70*(1), 177–179.

Federal Emergency Management Agency (FEMA). (n.d.). *The shelter-in-place pictogram guidance*. www.fema.gov/sites/default/files/documents/fema_shelter-in-place_guidance.pdf

GrowNYC. (2018, October 22). *GrowNYC's green book 2018*. Issue. https://issuu.com/grownyc/docs/grownyc_greenbook2018

Hester, J. L. (2017, October 27). The long tail of a storm. *CityLab*. www.citylab.com/environment/2017/10/sandy-5-years-later/544185/

Hormel Foods. (n.d.). What is SPAM? *SPAM*. www.spam.com/what-is-spam

IMDb. (n.d.). Contagion user reviews. *IMDb*. www.imdb.com/title/tt1598778/reviews/?ref_=ttrt_sa_3

Misdary, R. (2023, October 30). How an 8-acre green roof atop the Javits Center is boosting NYC's biodiversity. *Gothamist.* https://gothamist.com/news/how-an-8-acre-green-roof-atop-the-javits-center-is-boosting-nyc-biodiversity
Moena, B. (2006, March 9). Leavitt urges people, institutions to take precaution against flu. *Billings Gazette.* https://billingsgazette.com/news/state-and-regional/wyoming/leavitt-urges-people-institutions-to-take-precaution-against-flu/article_f9fc1a64-9f6e-5b86-9591-ce03f1bd4665.html
NYC Parks. (n.d.). *About green thumb.* https://www.nycgovparks.org/greenthumb/about
Osnos, E. (2017, January 22). Doomsday prep for the super-rich. *The New Yorker.* www.newyorker.com/magazine/2017/01/30/doomsday-prep-for-the-super-rich
Popescu-Roberts, E., Veltri, C., Lozoya, M., Agostini-Walesch, G., & Mitchell, J. C. (2022). Nonprescription fish antibiotics: Are they the same as those prescribed to humans? *JADA Foundational Science, 1.*
Schimmenti, A., Billieux, J., & Starcevic, V. (2020). The four horsemen of fear: An integrated model of understanding fear experiences during the COVID-19 pandemic. *Clinical Neuropsychiatry: Journal of Treatment Evaluation, 17*(2), 41–45.
Shamberg, M. (Producer), & Soderbergh, S. (Director). (2011). *Contagion* [motion picture]. Warner Bros.
Simonson, R. (2020, May 14). Canned cocktails in quarantine make mixing a one-step process. *The New York Times.* www.nytimes.com/2020/05/14/dining/drinks/canned-cocktails-coronavirus.html
Sperling, N. (2020, March 4). "Contagion," Steven Soderbergh's 2011 thriller, is climbing up the charts. *The New York Times.* www.nytimes.com/2020/03/04/business/media/coronavirus-contagion-movie.html
Terlep, S. (2021, January 2). Hand sanitizer sales jumped 600% in 2020. Purell maker bets against a post-pandemic collapse. *The Wall Street Journal.* www.wsj.com/articles/hand-sanitizer-sales-jumped-600-in-2020-purell-maker-bets-against-a-post-pandemic-collapse-11611311430
Zhang, S., Wu, S., Wu, Q., Durkin, D., & Marsiglia, F. (2021). Adolescent drug use initiation and transition into other drugs: A retrospective longitudinal examination across race/ethnicity. *Addictive Behaviors, 113.*

5

SETTLING IN AND SETTLING DOWN

Life During Lockdown

I often enjoy a favorite pastime of all New Yorkers. I like to complain about how much the city has changed. I even follow Jeremiah Moss's Instagram account called "Vanishing New York" so I can be outraged by the latest photos of the ruination of our city or to smile over the photos of free spirits and eccentrics who gather at Washington Square.[1] We all mourn losses as our city changes. No doubt, Gentle Reader, you are going through the catalogue of your favorite losses right now. (The subway token perhaps? I understand.) My biggest loss surprises even me. What do I miss about New York? I miss the Forbes Galleries that was once housed within the Forbes Building on Fifth Avenue (between 12th and 13th Streets). It was a hidden gem in my Greenwich Village neighborhood. Sometimes after visiting the Galleries, I would spot editor-in-chief Steve Forbes eating lunch at Joe Junior's on 11th Street (before the diner closed – another loss). We seemed to eat at the same time. We both even ordered the same hamburger. Steve always wore a free Forbes tie, the one that you would get as a gift for subscribing to the magazine. However, I am not certain that his cost-saving strategy worked, as the Forbes Galleries were shuttered when the company moved its headquarters to Jersey City in 2014.[2] As noted in a *New York Times* review of small museums in the city:

> Malcolm Forbes designed this enticingly escapist space in the ground floor of his magazine empire headquarters as a home for his fantastic collection of toy ships and soldiers, with very real famous manuscripts, a dozen Imperial Easter Eggs designed by Fabergé, and an art exhibition thrown in for good measure.
>
> *(Shepard, 1991)*

DOI: 10.4324/9781003400356-5

Never mind the 500 toys ships, the 12,000 soldiers, Abraham Lincoln's top hat, and Thomas Jefferson's desperate letter to his nephew in which the former president begs for money. Whenever I passed by and I had a few extra minutes, I would pop in to admire the earliest Monopoly game, thought to be from 1933.[3] The game board is actually circular and it comes with the first set of written rules. Forbes's father, Malcolm Forbes, is said to have collected early versions of the game due to his love of capitalism (*Antiques Trade Gazette*, 2011). Given his family's success, this interest makes sense. However, I find it curious that this land-trading game in which players make or lose pretend fortunes got its start during the Great Depression. I love playing Monopoly, but an interest in playing this game during a time of economic turmoil seems to be more complicated than amusement. Were people playing the game to try to gain a better sense of control or understanding of the crisis of their time? Did playing the game give people the chance to face their fears about the economic downturn? I do not think that the game was just escapism or play. It may have been providing players with some type of release.

In 2020, the Pandemic game seemed to offer a similar outlet. Released in 2008, Pandemic is a cooperative board game in which players are members of disease control teams. Played on a board with a map of the world, the objective is to work together to develop cures and to prevent outbreaks of four deadly diseases before they contaminate the globe. Much like life, the players all win or lose together. At the start of the COVID-19 pandemic, the game surged in popularity with over two million copies sold (Marshall, 2021).[4] Considered a favorite among doctors battling the disease, interest in the game moved "from curiosity to cathartic release to offering, in miniature, a finite version of our stricken world" (Jahromi, 2020, para. 1). Each player is a character important to protecting the population and finding cures. These characters include: Contingency Planner, Dispatcher, Medic, Operations Expert, Quarantine Specialist, Researcher, and Scientist. For me, playing Pandemic was unsettling because it served as a reminder of the reality of COVID-19; even if we discovered a vaccine for it, we really weren't solving all of the problems wrought by the virus. A vaccine or cure would only be the initial step. The game has no characters like a psychologist or sociologist to analyze and help fix the long-term consequences of a pandemic for individuals or society. What about a pandemic's profound impact on employment, mental health, or education? However, in the game, there is one event card that speaks to the possible role of preppers in slowing down the spread of disease. In the game, a card called "Resilient Population" can be played as a temporary buffer between the Infect and Intensify steps of an epidemic.

As a game, Pandemic cannot really address the sense of loneliness and the fears that ordinary people experienced during lockdown. Its elite disease control team would have no use for a character called "New Yorker Trapped in Tiny Apartment." Yet, such a character might provide a way to think about the complex emotions caused by the pandemic. How individuals cope with their anxiety and fears determines society's resilience in responding to a catastrophe, according to Schimmenti et al. (2020), because those emotions affect our sense of agency and behaviors. By addressing their fears and learning survival skills, were New Yorkers practicing self-reliance to better protect themselves? Were New York preppers able to better protect themselves during the pandemic?

This chapter discusses the challenges and success of New York Preppers' sheltering-in-place experiences. First, the chapter explores the response of preppers to the management of the pandemic by government. Next, it looks at the importance during the pandemic of preparedness strategies such the significance of the prepper closet to households and the value of networks to secure information and resources. Lastly, the chapter examines the challenges experienced by preppers. Like so many other New Yorkers living through the pandemic, preppers in one cramped dwelling were suddenly faced with the challenge of accommodating and balancing many facets of life, such as eating, playing, sleeping, and working from home. Many individuals, especially parents, also had to assume potentially new and unfamiliar roles, including teacher for remote learning, doctor, therapist, and entertainer. New York preppers benefited greatly during the pandemic from their training; however, they discovered that they had overly focused on the wrong disaster scenario. While they had learned sheltering-in-place strategies, they had focused on bushcraft – wilderness survival skills – because of the assumption that they would have to leave the city.

For most New York City preppers, the pandemic was not their first test. Rather than having to imagine possible scenarios, they had already learned preparedness and survival skills based on their direct experience of the city's recent history of disasters and crises, as discussed in Chapter 2. In the weeks before New York was shuttered for COVID-19, Jason Charles, the leader of the NYCPN, felt confident about his group's ability to withstand the pandemic based on its members' training and their ownership of personal protective equipment. As noted in the best-selling *The Ultimate Prepper's Survival Bible*, the goal of prepping is to "prepare yourself, your family, and your home before an emergency situation arises. This will ensure that your family is as safe as possible during a crisis" (Pearson, 2023). Most New York City preppers were prepared for the pandemic by the end of January. This readiness is significant because it reflects their level of alertness to media reports and their firm belief in needing to protect their families. By adhering to their practice of self-reliance, they believed that they could potentially decrease their risk of contracting the virus as they had their own protective equipment and supplies. Rather than waiting for guidance or supplies that might never be provided by the government, they could act swiftly and independently to support their families and communities. The pandemic, especially the first phase, proved to be a critical test for these urban preppers, which demonstrated the strengths of their philosophy of preparedness and their survival skills.

Most important, the mismanagement of the pandemic response by all three levels of the government – federal, state, and city – reinforced their belief in self-reliance. For urban preppers, the government's failure to enact a clear response to the pandemic reaffirmed their core belief: the government was not coming to save them. Instead, they would have to rely on themselves and their local networks. One Brooklyn African-American female prepper[5] argued that the federal government's inability to manage the COVID crisis resulted in "a game of 'Whac-A-Mole' where problems related to the virus and confusion keep popping up." These urban preppers expressed concerns similar to other Americans about the management of the pandemic such as the lack of presidential leadership, the shortage of protective equipment, and economic instability. As Wright (2022, p. 114) notes, these policy problems compounded the danger of existing "socially created vulnerabilities" such as healthcare inequalities and overcrowded housing.

Like other Americans, preppers lamented the ineptitude of the government and the subsequent loss of life. In response to these failures, they stressed the importance of continued self-reliance. Urban preppers also utilized social media platforms such as Instagram and Facebook to provide tips about sheltering in place and protection against the virus. Beginning in January, Instagram posts from Jason Charles, leader of the New York City Prepper's Network, included information such as news updates about the spread of COVID-19, a fact sheet on "How to Stop the Spread in NYC," and an interview with an Italian who was sheltering in place (Italy adopted a shelter-in-place policy earlier than the United States) as well as funny memes like a photo of Forrest Gump with the caption, "And, just like that. . . . Everyone Stopped Making Fun of Preppers." The leaders also sometimes provided advice or correction to others who posted on social media. For example, I posted a picture on social media of a clever sign promoting the wearing of masks. Jason responded quickly to remind me that, while the message may have been clever, the mask pictured would have been ineffective in protecting against COVID-19.

To assist his 153-member group, Marlon, a seasoned prepper and leader of the UOS, led online meetings and workshops designed to improve sheltering-in-place skills, such as extending the serving size and shelf life of food. For example, UOS members were provided with a PowerPoint talk designed to offer storage and food advice for better prepper closet management. During the online meeting, photographs of two-liter bottles filled with sugar or rice (with oxygen absorbers) were introduced as inexpensive, smart storage solutions. Lists of "Zero-Prep" foods, like read-to-eat canned meals and protein bars, were also distributed as preparation reminders for members in the event of a blackout. Powdered milk and instant coffee were also recommended (Clear signs of the apocalypse to me).

Another long-time Brooklyn prepper's direct experience involving the shortage of personal protective equipment reinforced this lack of trust in the government's ability to meet the needs of citizens.[6] In late March, this prepper posted an extra N95 mask for sale on an e-commerce site that facilitates consumer-to-consumer sales. As she recounted:

> I ended up giving it away. I gave it to a doctor working in a New York Pediatrics Department. He said that the hospital had nothing for them so they were all searching and trying to buy their own stuff. How could I take his money? The man cares for children. I felt terrible. We all knew that there were going to be shortages, that it was going to be bad, but it happened so quickly. A doctor searching around for his own supplies. I wanted to do something nice. I gave him a roll of toilet paper too. I mean, I wanted him to know that we are all in this together. Such a crazy thing. Toilet paper.

For Ron, another experienced urban prepper, government policies implemented to fairly allocate resources were an important indicator of security. He compared government interventions in aiding residents during the pandemic to government policies enacted during the aftermath of Hurricane Sandy. He recalled:

> In Hurricane Sandy, there was a rationing of gas, there was a policy to deal with that shortage. Now, citizens have no confidence in government. They are fearing the worst-case scenarios about everything. How has the government helped with the pandemic? Sure, they partially helped the economy with the stimulus package but that was after the virus had spread and after the first layoffs.

Throughout the height of the pandemic, New York City preppers sought to bolster their safety by participating in information and resource networks. In contrast to the stereotype that casts preppers as suspicious loners, many of the city's preppers have strong social networks and are often members of civic or parochial groups. For example, prior to COVID's spread to New York, urban preppers used information networks to exchange information about the potential threat of COVID and discussed their respective approaches to sheltering in place. During virtual meetings of both the NYCPN and the UOS, members exchanged information about the impact of the pandemic in their respective areas and networked for needed supplies (such as extra masks or disinfectant for new members). Ron attributed his participation in social networks to his success in sheltering in place:

> Working within groups and networks made me do better than an average person. This is about staying ahead of the curve. I always try to talk to

> people. You never know what you are going to learn and how you could help each other. In the fall, I spent a lot of time concentrating on wilderness survival skills. After talking to and exchanging ideas with other preppers, I realized I needed to switch gears. By January, I was finishing up my preps. I have connections to get most things. I also have an agreement with my neighbor to look out for each other.

New York City preppers fielded questions in person, by phone, and by text from neighbors about preparations for the pandemic, gave supplies such as masks and gloves to neighbors in need, and organized or participated in neighborhood networks to deliver medication and groceries to elderly or disabled residents. In response to his new popularity, Marlon explained, "For years, I have been the weirdo. Now, everyone is calling me like I am their best friend. Hey, I am just glad that they are finally listening to me." LaChelle, a longtime prepper from Brooklyn, observed:

> We are vindicated – not that we wanted to be. We want to help people. That's what this is about. You can't survive without being a community. That's why our country is having so much trouble, we all need to be working together. Everyone reached out to me. I texted supplies lists to my college friends. I worked with my family and friends. Everybody had questions about what to do.

For New York City preppers, knowledge of sheltering-in-place skills and maintaining a prepper closet were key assets during lockdown. By relying on their skills and their stores, the city's preppers were better protected from challenges such as unfamiliarity with staying home to avoid danger, the lack of protection against the spread of COVD-19, the possibility of food shortages, the lack of medical supplies, the sudden challenges of unemployment, and the absence of support during lockdown. Did New York City preppers bear extraordinary burdens like other people who stayed in the city? Yes. However, their knowledge of sheltering-in-place skills helped them to adapt more quickly. As discussed in Chapter 4, New York City preppers already had "prepper closets," stocked up for use in any type of disaster. Unlike non-preppers who had to learn about the importance of storing items such as shelf-stable food and medical supplies, and then secure these items within just a few weeks, New York City preppers were already familiar with the knowledge and had supplies. Therefore, these preppers could quickly adapt to the unique features of a pandemic even though their preparations were based on their experience of different challenges. For example, in response to the early warning about the pandemic, New York City preppers could quickly pivot to expand their provisions to include extra masks (mainly N95), face shields, disposable gloves, disinfectant, and hand sanitizer, (including the ingredients to make it). Furthermore, after concluding that power outages were not common in areas of China that had already been hit hard by the pandemic, some urban preppers decided the same would apply in the United States and purchased deep freezers to stock up on meat and other frozen items.

Lastly, New York City preppers were already practicing homesteading skills. They had been canning and preserving food for years, while other Americans, rushing to try it, were causing a shortage of Mason jars. New York City preppers were reminding people to also search for jars at places like craft and thrift stores. Rather than becoming unsettled, the New York City preppers were settling in. I suspect that the Mason jar shortage may also have been sparked not just by an interest in preserving fruit in water baths or repurposing them as drinking glasses or candle holders or terrariums. Instead, Mason jars are important symbols in American culture. Their use seems to represent both control and comfort in one's home. As Kelly (2015) writes, "Mason jars suggest resistance to the mass production of food and culture; they emphasize the values of self-sufficiency and community. Mason jars, with their pleasing shape and transparency, suggest a kind of wholesome luxury."[7]

Although ready.gov (Department of Homeland Security, 2023) suggests that Americans keep several-days' supply of food and water on hand, urban preppers interviewed had at least one-month's stock of nonperishable food. At the start of the pandemic, policy experts and food distributors did not expect a food shortage in New York; however, there was concern about food-insecure populations and the increasing numbers of unemployed residents (Lederer, 2020). Before the pandemic, 1.2 million New Yorkers were food insecure, including vulnerable groups such as senior citizens and school-age children who qualify for free or reduced-priced meals (The Mayor's Office for Food Policy, 2019). With the unemployment rate near 20% in July 2020 (McGeehan, 2020), many more New Yorkers struggled to feed their families. According to City Harvest, one of the largest emergency food distributors in the city, nearly 12 million New Yorkers visited pantries in its network from March through August of that year, roughly three million more that the same period in 2019 (Stewart & Heisler, 2020). Meeting the increased demand was made more challenging by the closure of many food pantries due to labor shortages caused by the pandemic.[8] Many food bank volunteers were senior citizens who were at greater risk of contracting COVID-19. For example, the Food Bank for New York City typically supplies about 1,000 sites, either food pantries or soup kitchens, with groceries (Aridi, 2020). By mid-April, 40% of the sites had closed due to the outbreak. As expressed by a *New York Times* reader in the comments section about an article on the city's high unemployment rate, "Life in New York I suspect will never be the same. Poor people will bear the most pain as they always do. Seeing people lining up for hours at food pantries is heartbreaking" (McGeehan, 2020).

Through networking, New York City preppers also worked to provide food and needed supplies to more vulnerable senior citizens in their communities who struggled at home. Their efforts ranged from responding to phone calls from elderly neighborhoods seeking help to organizing groups of helpful neighbors. Tracy, a Queens prepper, recounted on Facebook her efforts to help an elderly friend:

> My neighbor was sick with COVID in her home for 3 weeks. She is a senior and lives alone. Every day, I walked 10 blocks to bring her food. I prepped in January for 3 months of food, so I had plenty to share. There was supposed to be a food bank in NYC that would deliver food to her but they never came.

A Manhattan prepper organized a Facebook page for his apartment building so that neighbors could share news and help one another while sheltering in place. Through communicating via Facebook and texting, participating residents coordinated grocery runs and pharmacy pick-ups to assist the senior citizens who remained in the building. Via grocery store websites and Instacart memberships, some preppers even arranged grocery deliveries for elderly relatives and friends who lived out of state. As someone who researches preppers, I also responded to calls from individuals trying to figure out how to secure items that were sometimes out of stock. Some requests were less serious than others. My friend and I had chuckled over a young mother's worry about being unable to find disposable diapers for her newborn. The lack of disposable diapers in the proper size is inconvenient, no doubt. However, she had not heard of cloth diapers. ("You mean that you actually wash them and use them again?" Yes.)

Through having prepper closets, these New Yorkers were better protected against the possibility of hunger. Prior to lockdown, they were able to avoid panic buying. After lockdown, in response to minor shortages at grocery stores, urban preppers relied on their prepping closets to replace items that were out of stock such as yeast for baking or a preferred brand of spaghetti sauce. As the death rate continued to escalate in the city from late March through mid-April, grocery-store trips were viewed as risky and resulted in overwhelming grocery delivery services which were unable to meet the demand. Therefore, New York City preppers "shopped" their prepper closets. Given New York's rapid economic downturn, some preppers' amply stocked closets also served as a vital buffer against hunger. For an older White Brooklyn couple who had only started prepping in 2018,[9] their prepper closet with one month's supply of food helped them to weather a job loss early in the pandemic. As the husband said, "Only one of us has a job that allows us to work virtually. The repair shop where I worked folded almost immediately. We were down to one income. Having a stockpile of food and everyday stuff took the edge off. We could stretch things out. It's helped us not to immediately deplete our savings. Otherwise, we would've gone through it like a buzzsaw."

Urban preppers were also able to rely on "go money" to cushion against lost wages. "Go money" is cash saved by preppers for use during disaster. This money is usually hidden in a secret location within a home – not always within a safe – for immediate retrieval if the prepper has to leave the home in search of safety. The expectation is that "go money" will used on the road after a prepper has "bugged out." During interviews, some preppers were willing to disclose that they kept amounts ranging from $1,000 to $5,000 as "go money." Erik, a young White male prepper from the East Village who worked as a bartender shared that his "go money" was useful in meeting expenses after his place of employment closed.

> I didn't think twice about it. That's what 'go money' is for – to help save you. I used it to cover my bills for a while. My girlfriend and I had just moved in together. I didn't want to be a sponge. It helped out. It also helped her understand the value of prepping. Not just monetary value. The value of planning ahead.

Erik reported having $2,200 stashed as "go money" and around $900 in his savings account.

Prepper closets were also used to store protective gear to guard against COVID-19. Most urban preppers had an array of protective equipment such as N95 masks, face shields, disposable gloves, disinfectants, hand sanitizer, and even hazmat suits. Preppers reported wearing protective gear and regular clothing that covered their entire bodies when outside of their homes. These precautions were also taken early on in the pandemic and without a government directive. Some urban preppers who traveled by plane for work began wearing face masks in January, months before the airline industry announced that face masks were recommended for travel in May. As LaChelle noted:

> I couldn't believe that they told people that they didn't need to wear masks. You are trying to avoid catching a deadly virus. How could you not wear a mask? I stopped listening and did all that I could do to protect myself whenever I left home.

Beyond wearing protective equipment, urban preppers also set up decontamination stations near their front doors to disinfect incoming packages like mail, newspapers, and deliveries, and to remove clothing and footwear that had been worn outside.

New York City preppers also benefited from having additional medicine and first aid supplies for sheltering in place. Given their preparations, they did not need to rush around to various pharmacies to buy needed over-the-counter medicine. In addition, many preppers avoided stress by contacting their doctors in advance of lockdown for prescription refills. They also had different types of antibiotics on hand in case of emergency. With first aid training, these preppers felt prepared to treat minor injuries at home rather than risking a visit to an urgent care clinic or an emergency room.

However, New York City preppers still had to contend with family members who contracted mild cases of COVID-19. As part of their preparedness training and before the news of a possible pandemic, many preppers had already developed plans on how to "quarantine" family members at home. After learning about the dangers of COVID-19, some preppers had even purchased oximeters to test the oxygen intake of a family member who contracted COVID-19.

Typical plans involved quarantining an ill family member in a bedroom with food, medicine, and fresh linens delivered outside the door on a tray. Disposable glasses, plates, napkins, and utensils would be used and then discarded after every meal. Dirty linens would be placed in a trash bag next to the tray. Contact would be maintained via calling or texting so that the ill person didn't need to shout or poke their head out of the door. Items would be delivered or picked up at the door by a designated family member who would be wearing a mask and gloves. In most cases, it seemed that the mother or wife would be the primary care taker. If weather permitted, the bedroom windows would be opened for fresh air. Disinfectant spray would be used periodically in the bedroom and throughout the home. If there was only one bathroom in the apartment, the bathroom would be disinfected after use by the primary caregiver. If well enough, the ill family member would monitor and report their oxygen intake. Otherwise, the primary caretaker would assume this responsibility.

A Bronx prepper family relied on their plan to care for a family member who contracted COVID-19. Shortly before lockdown, the husband and father, Al, caught COVID-19 at his job, which required face-to-face contact with the public. According to Annette, the mother and wife, their plan of confining her husband to a bedroom was effective. For her, having a plan in advance reduced the anxiety and stress of trying to figure out how to best care for a person and how to protect their children at the last minute. As her husband's primary caregiver, Annette explained, "the craziness of receiving text messages from him in the bedroom" adding that "it was a very stressful time because he was sick for weeks." Later, Annette also contracted COVID. Echoing the plight of other primary caregivers, she shared that she did not exactly receive the same level of care and attention that she had provided or relief from household responsibilities. According to a national study of gender division of labor during lockdown (Waddell et al., 2021), women completed more of the parenting and household tasks, while men spent more time on their jobs and on personal time; males who were the primary caregivers before the pandemic also experienced the same unequal division of labor.

For many New Yorkers in romantic relationships, sheltering-in-place meant sometimes facing the challenges that might arise from spending too much time together in close quarters. However, for some New Yorkers who had just started relationship before the pandemic, sheltering-in-place created a sense of longing and a search for ways to maintain the connection. For example, Ehsaan, a Queens prepper of three years in his late twenties, faced the challenge of dating a girl only to be separated just 2 months after they had met. As he explains:

> There was no way that we could risk seeing each other. Her grandparents live with her and my brother is a doctor. We had to figure out how to spend time together besides just talking or texting. We looked for things to do together. We played games. We watched movies. We even did art projects together. I really missed her, but we knew that this would allow us to really get to know each other. After lockdown, our first date was sitting outside, in her backyard. Because of our families, we still had to be so careful.

In a lively *Huffington Post* interview, I was asked to name my favorite songs about the apocalypse. To understand the perception of preppers in American culture, I have spent time researching representations of the apocalypse in American culture so I am familiar with this song category. When it comes to expressing longing while sheltering-in-place, The Postal Service's "We Will Become Silhouettes" (2005) is jarring and oddly beautiful. Until Ehsaan shared his heartache with me, I really didn't sense the full power of the song's lyrics: "I've got a cupboard with cans of food/Filtered water and pictures of you/And I'm not coming out until this is all over."[10]

While it is useful to learn sheltering-in-place strategies to ensure that one's family's needs are met during a pandemic, these skills did not completely prepare urban preppers for the many mental and physical challenges of everyday life during lockdown. Beyond providing information and needed supplies, networks also offered urban preppers encouragement and support as residents sheltered in place in the American epicenter of the virus. During an April NYCPN online meeting about sheltering in place, Jason, the group's leader, encouraged members not just to look at prepping for stability but also to turn to whatever sense of spirituality they had to help them stay strong as the city's death rate escalated. At the time, I had been a member of the network for roughly 5 years as a participant-observer. During that time, I had attended many meetings, excursions, and workshops led by Jason. I had observed him during moments of happiness and satisfaction – over the group's mastery of a skill, for example – and in moments of pressure such as when, on an outdoor excursion, he administered first aid to a member who had severely cut his hand and then drove the member to the hospital several miles from the campsite. I have even heard him share the story, in a matter-of-fact way, of being a first responder on September 11th and seeing marauders arrive to search the dead for money and jewelry.[11] This April meeting was the first time that I saw him deeply concerned. When sharing his suggestion to seek support, he paused and shook his head in a moment of disbelief. His reaction was understandable. From March through April 3, New York City lost 2,172 residents to COVID-19 (NYT, n.d.).

As the pandemic continued, I noticed that Jason began to emphasize the number of people who had recovered rather than those who had died, as his interest focused on maintaining morale. On Facebook, he posted a table of COVID-19 cases that provided both the number of deaths and number of recoveries. He reminded members to focus on the high number of recoveries. He also posted on Instagram that he "had a disdain for the media and politicians because they were trying to scare everyone by always talking about deaths and playing to fears rather than talking about the number of people who recovered."

During this same time period, I spoke with Marlon, the leader of the UOS about his experiences as a leader in the prepping community. Before launching the group, Marlon was a leader in the NYCPN. For me, as well as many other preppers, Marlon has been an important mentor. He is a skilled and compassionate leader. He's generous with his advice, support and heart. He shared with me that, as the leader of the UOS, he fielded calls from preppers and non-preppers needing to talk about a range of pressures caused by the pandemic such as the tragic passing of loved ones, job loss, and frustrations related to sheltering in place. Marlon is usually upbeat and ready to share a quick story or funny observation to express his point. However, in this conversation, Marlon spoke slower and softer. He shared a bit about "the heaviness" of a talk that he had just had with a member for whom "things were really tough." I could hear the sadness in his voice as he talked about how he had carefully planned out the mission of the group and how it was intended to teach people vital prepping knowledge and skills. He explained that he didn't think about how members might need this type of support and that he now realized its importance. To address the needs of members, Marlon began work on incorporating stress-reduction strategies into his classes on sheltering in place. He also began posting positive and encouraging posts on Instagram like, "The same boiling water that softens the potato hardens the egg. It's about what you're made of, not the circumstances." Underneath this particular post, he added reminded viewers that "we have all been pushed right to the brink . . . and we did not fall."

The pandemic exaggerated the stressors of ordinary life. Before lockdown, parents worried about how well their children were doing in school. Suddenly, school and home collapsed into one. During lockdown, most New Yorkers with children, including preppers, struggled with their unexpected roles as teachers once schools moved online. As Julia explained:

> I never really expected this. I always expected that if something really bad happened in the city we would have to bug out, that we'd be rushing somewhere and outside, trying to reach safety. I never thought that we would be stuck inside . . . that the stress and the crazy would be about things like trying to schedule teaching and learning time for my three kids on a computer. Honestly, I thought that this was going to be about not having technology.

Across the country, parents working from home struggled with remote learning problems including learning different meeting platforms, trying to relearn and then teach to their children something they had long forgotten, and cajoling older children into submitting assignments (Harris & Jones, 2020). A Manhattan father[12] of an elementary school student and prepper of six years remarked on remote learning:

> I was at work all the time. I was exhausted like everyone else. I alternated between taking meetings and teaching my son. As he worked his way through the lesson, I was on the iPad searching for enrichment materials to explain things to him. We were a tag-team. For next year, I'm going to try to find teacher manuals to help us through.

With New York City schools online by late April, children without access to a computer and a broadband connection were unable to engage in virtual learning. Before the pandemic, this limitation created a "homework gap" that impacted students' ability to complement their school-based education with online resources at home, complete assignments, and access resources about college opportunities (U.S. Congress Joint Economic Committee, 2017). The pandemic exacerbated this "digital divide," as these students were completely denied access to online learning. Given the swift spread of the virus, New York's Department of Education quickly implemented a distance-learning program with only limited planning for its 1.1 million students, providing 475,000 devices, including tablets and laptops to students (Gould, 2020). In addition to the challenges of online learning, the pandemic also impacted family life for New Yorkers by eliminating or greatly reducing the use of parks and public spaces. To prevent the contraction of COVID-19, parents were reluctant to use these spaces, and then, once the city closed the playgrounds in April, unable to take their children outside to play and enjoy a sense of freedom and fresh air. Few New Yorkers have the luxury of outdoor space at home, so park closures were particularly hard. Some urban preppers recognized that the lack of public space would be challenging for their children, so they prepared in advance. A Manhattan mother and prepper with two elementary school children created what she referred to as an Activity Closet:

> I made some space in my bedroom closet to store new games, books, and craft kits for the pandemic. When their spirits seemed low or I felt that we needed to change things up, I would sometimes bring out something new. Pick-up Sticks was a great crowd pleaser. We also did fun workout routines that we found on YouTube. In our apartment, going stir crazy was contagious. Trust me, they had plenty of fights, but we managed okay.

Like so many New Yorkers, urban preppers have come to recognize that long-term sheltering in place requires not only a careful work/life balance for all members of the household, but dedicated time for enjoyment and discovery, even in cramped quarters.

For urban preppers, the pandemic has been a lesson in endurance that has allowed them to test their mettle during a real-life disaster. Given their interest in protecting their families against disasters like pandemics, urban preppers were prepared to prevent the spread of the virus much earlier than other New Yorkers. All preppers that I interviewed reported being ready for the pandemic by the end of January, nearly 2 months before New York's shelter-in-place order on March 22. Prior to the pandemic, they already owned personal protective equipment and were familiar with the correct use of each item, such as wearing properly fitting N95 masks. These urban preppers were able to refrain from panic buying to prepare for sheltering in place during the pandemic, because they had already stockpiled food and essential items in their prepper closets. All interviewed preppers indicated having at least a 30-day supply of provisions. Prior to and throughout the pandemic, these urban preppers also participated in information-and-resource-exchange networks to prepare and assist others during the pandemic. Furthermore, many urban preppers served their respective communities by teaching neighbors how to prepare for the pandemic and helping to secure needed supplies by donating supplies or providing a contact for the particular item.

While these urban preppers had a strong foundation for successfully preparing to shelter in place, they did not anticipate the unique challenges of staying in their homes for such an extended time period. Some preppers had expected that a great disaster would most likely involve leaving the city. Others also imagined that they would probably not have access to technology such as the Internet and laptops during such a crisis. Therefore, urban preppers came to recognize that long-term sheltering in place requires a careful work/life balance for all members of the household. Remote learning was particularly taxing for employed parents as they juggled helping their children to complete their schooling while simultaneously meeting their own job responsibilities. Furthermore, this strain was compounded when families competed for computer use and broadband access.

Like most New Yorkers who sheltered in place for weeks, these urban preppers also struggled with the difficulties of living in a city devoid of its vibrancy and the opportunity to connect with others outside of one's home. Echoing the sentiments of other preppers, LaChelle said, "I've learned how difficult it is to live in a real-life lockdown, I really missed my family and my friends, especially my cousins. This has made me think about long-term community building. We are stronger together."

After the lockdown ended, New York City preppers did not spend time congratulating themselves on their level of preparedness. As with other disasters in the city, they learned from their direct experiences and began preparing for another round of infections and possible lockdown. To prepare for a possible second wave of the virus in the fall, these urban preppers sought to replenish their supplies and made some modifications to their sheltering-in-place plans. Most urban preppers had placed orders for additional protective equipment such as masks by the spring to ensure delivery by September. Expecting that they would need to shelter in place for a prolonged period amidst a collapsing economy, some urban preppers worked to ensure their prepper closets contained provisions to last up to a year. This step would require securing additional space such as a storage facility. Anticipating that school would still be online, many urban preppers invested in new technology, buying additional laptops or tablets. To improve the ability of family members to access the Internet simultaneously without difficulties, some preppers boosted their connection speeds. Urban preppers also sought to maximize the use of space in their apartment by rearranging existing furniture, or purchasing new furniture to provide designated work, learning, or entertainment spaces. A few preppers started working together to develop plans to create a large survival cache, a large storage facility space that functions as a supply house, to support their families and those needing assistance.

After lockdown, many other Americans also considered ways to improve the lives of their families in the event of subsequent waves of the pandemic. Recall the shortage of items that facilitated both work and learning at home, like desks, laptops, and printers, for example. However, in their commitment to self-reliance and trying to plan for even greater hardships as the pandemic continued, New York preppers formed an unexpected and very valuable alliance. The Hudson Valley Prepper & Survival group was founded in 2020. Michael Kaleb, the group's founder, shares prepping and survival skills through live streams, live events, and social media. Founded in 2020, this Hudson Valley prepper group has 1,156 members (roughly 60% men and 40% women). The majority of members are from the Hudson Valley, with ages ranging from 25 to 64. Most members live in the Hudson Valley area and in the city.[13] Given their mutual commitments to self-reliance and their proximity to one another, the two group leaders began developing a regional network of preppers who live in the city and preppers who in the Hudson Valley to help one another in future crises.

I was very curious about the first appearance of the Hudson Valley group's founder at an online meeting of the NYCPN. He was definitely not an urban prepper. He looked like the Brawny man sitting outside on the steps of his big front porch in the Catskills. At one point, he even lit a cigarette. He did not speak; however, he nodded thoughtfully as Jason told the group:

> If you don't have community, you aren't going to make it. A 60-year-old asshole isn't going to change, but there could be a recognition of advantages that you would have by working together. The goal is to find like-minded people, to find your tribe.

Initially, it seemed the concept was only an extended network to exchange resources and information between preppers in and outside of the city. However, the discussion moved beyond ideas like meeting to exchange goods or hiding joint caches along designated routes. The concept also included forming small communities for survival. Michael strongly believes that building community is the key to surviving disaster. In our conversation and in his YouTube Live Streams, he encourages people to talk with their neighbors because "neighbors are your best defense and a disaster is not the time to finally start talking to one another." According to Michael, there are misperceptions about city people who may come to the Hudson Valley following a disaster:

> People believe that hordes of people from the city are going to come here, like grasshoppers and devour all that we have. But that is not true. Different communities will need to band together and cast out the bad people. It is going to take a lot of hands and effort to clean up the land and get going. There are going to be good people who have a skill set but have not prepared. They are going to be a great asset and loyal to the community.

This interconnection holds tremendous significance for two reasons. First, this type of community could strengthen the potential force of local resilience with increased knowledge, resources and labor. Second, the development of such a community would be created independently from government relief efforts. Its main advantage is that it would sidestep government mismanagement and inefficiencies in meeting the needs of citizens. Therefore, this type of community may provide the critical advantages of adaptation and flexibility. Jason referred to such a collective as a "sustaining community." When asked if this type of community could be considered a commune or compound, they rejected both categories. However, they had different notions about the mission of this type of community. Michael perceives that they would be small communities of people working together to survive and also networking with other communities as needed.

Jason takes a harder tack in conceptualizing a "sustaining community," which would be governed by "input from everyone" and support public resources like a community garden and provisions. However, for Jason, a "sustaining community" could be thought of as "developing a parallel society big enough where government doesn't want to fuck with us because there is going to be a fight." Both leaders encourage the cross-pollination of their groups to help make connections for designing preparedness strategies and community planning. In speaking with Michael about community-building, my mind turned to urban citizenship and the importance of the locals. As he shared the origins of his idea, his sense of connection and compassion rang true:

> As friends started to move away, I didn't want them to feel like they were left out. I want to help people connect. With over 1,000 members in my group [from various places], I hope that they can find someone in their community. The locals should rule. Let people talk and deal with each other. There are good people everywhere. I want people to find their tribe. We have to learn from each other.

I also considered Jason's edgier perspective. He seemed interested in relying on the community not just to sustain one another but also to shield one another from government intervention. Jason's conservative position and his disgust in what he views as government ineptitude has been long standing. After all, he founded the NYCPN in an effort to help people protect themselves as he believed that the government would be overwhelmed if required to respond to a catastrophe. As the pandemic continued, I came to understand his perspective better. As a member of New York Fire Department, Jason would be required to take a vaccine once it was developed. When the vaccine became available, he refused to take it. Jason felt that "the science wasn't there. The research was too fast and false. Plus, this was something for people with weaker immune systems to worry about, not people like me." Rather than complying with the vaccine mandate, Jason retired from the New York Fire Department.

Embedded in their respective ideas about establishing a community in the country and returning to a simpler form of life is "a myth functioning as memory" (Williams, 1975). In this imagined rural-urban divide, life in the country is thought to be pure and removed from social and economic changes. Conversely, the city is the nexus of capitalist greed, vice and alienation. However, this split is false. Both the country and the city hold many meanings and possibilities. These areas are not isolated from one another. Rather, the city and the country are not only linked by ideas and experiences but by factors such as economic interests and power relations (Williams,

1975). It is worth noting that in Yael Oved's (1988) classic history of American communes, a major challenge to maintaining a new communitarian life has been the difficulty that members had in leaving behind the outside world. The unwillingness to abandon their previous way of life was often the primary reason for disbandment.

In my last book, I found that, although preppers trained together, they did not necessarily plan to *survive* together. Typically, a prepper learns survival skills to better protect his/her/their family. Therefore, preppers plan to bug out with family members and/or friends, not members of the group. Given their different locations within the city, members would also plan to leave the city via different routes. Sometimes, there would be discussions about meeting up with others. A few preppers may have made secret agreements about meeting at a safe house;[14] however, this information was not shared within the group. As my research with preppers has continued, I have discovered that preppers whom I assumed would be bugging out together, did not necessarily do so. Therefore, the idea of planning a "sustained community" may be the next chapter in the prepping philosophy of self-reliance. The sense of the Local is becoming even more intertwined with the sense of Self. Tonight, when scrolling through Instagram, I saw that Jason posted a clip of a dilapidated and abandoned hospital or insane asylum (its location was listed as "nowhere"). As he toured the graffiti-covered building, he asked viewers, "What is your opinion on turning an insane asylum or abandoned hospital into a prepper community? Could you do something good with this or would you pass?" Viewers seemed divided on the question. The best comment came from lastprepperstanding:

> Spending the calories to fix that place up and build a community during SHTF no . . . doing prior sure especially if you can get the people who will be a part of the community to restore it together . . . that would be a great way to strengthen the bond of the community and really get people to take ownership.

Notes

1 For a discussion of the impact of the 21st century on New York, see Moss's book of the same name, Vanishing New York (2018).
2 In 2010, the building was purchased by New York University with a five-year occupancy agreement.
3 For an interesting history of the game's creation, see Pilon (2016).
4 The game's inventor, Matt Leacock, is now designing a similar game called Climate Crisis.
5 Name withheld and no name assigned at request.
6 Name withheld and no name assigned at request.
7 I am reminded of a story that my older friend once shared about her mother. In the 1950s, her mother was the first woman in the neighborhood to buy an automatic

dishwasher. This was surprising as her family's income was very modest in comparison to their neighbors. Her wealthier neighbor came over to inspect the new appliance. In a moment of jealousy, the neighbor asked, "How does it clean your fine China?" To which, my friend's mother replied: "It cleans my Mason jars just fine."

8 For a concise analysis of the impacts of COVID-19 on food banks such as the effects on operations and distribution, see Byrne and Just (2022). For a critique of the "hunger industrial complex," see Fisher (2017).

9 Names withheld and no name assigned at request.

10 The song can be found at The Postal Service – We Will Become Silhouettes [OFFICIAL VIDEO] – YouTube. www.youtube.com/watch?v=0rKC7ElkTUQ

11 In prepper discourse, people who are unprepared and who are on the hunt for resources like food and water are referred to as "zombies."

12 Name withheld and no name assigned at request.

13 However, there are also 18 members from other countries including four Canadians.

14 Given my research on prepping, I am often asked if I have a safe house. [Insert answer here.]

References

Antiques Trade Gazette. (2011, February 21). Earliest surviving "official" monopoly set makes $120,000. www.antiquestradegazette.com/news/2011/earliest-surviving-official-monopoly-set-makes-120-000/

Aridi, S. (2020). Facing food insecurity on the front lines. *The New York Times*. www.nytimes.com/2020/04/10/neediest-cases/feeding-america-food-banks-coronavirus.html

Byrne, A. T., & Just, D. R. (2022). Impacts of COVID-19 on food banks. *Choices (Ames, Iowa)*, *37*, 7.

Department of Homeland Security. (2023, August 4). Build a kit. *ready.gov*. www.ready.gov/kit

Fisher, A., & Jayaraman, S. (2017). *Big hunger: The unholy alliance between corporate America and anti-hunger groups*. The MIT Press.

Gould, J. (2020). NYC education department can't say how many students are getting live instruction through remote learning. *Gothamist*. https://gothamist.com/news/nyc-education-department-cant-say-how-many-students-are-getting-live-instruction-through-remote-learning

Harris, A., & Jones, M. (2020). COVID 19 – school leadership in disruptive times. *School Leadership & Management*, *40*(4), 243–247.

Jahromi, N. (2020, July 27). The board-game series for the age of coronavirus. *The New Yorker*. www.newyorker.com/culture/culture-desk/pandemic-the-board-game-series-for-the-age-of-the-coronavirus

Kelly, A. (2015, September 24). The mason jar, reborn. *The Atlantic*. www.theatlantic.com/technology/archive/2015/09/mason-jar-history/403762/

Lederer, A., Hoban, M., Lipson, S., Zhou, S., & Eisenberg, D. (2020). More than inconvenienced: The unique needs of U.S. college students during the COVID-19 pandemic. *Sage Journals*, *48*(1), 14–19.

Marshall, A. (2021, March 25). His game made beating a pandemic fun. Can he do it for climate change? *The New York Times*. www.nytimes.com/2021/03/25/arts/matt-leacock-climate-crisis-pandemic.html

The Mayor's Office for Food Policy. (2019). Food policy report 2019. *NYC.gov*. www.nyc.gov/assets/foodpolicy/downloads/pdf/Food-Policy-Report-2019.pdf

McGeehan, P. (2020). A million jobs lost: A "heart attack" for the N.Y.C. economy. *The New York Times*. Retrieved July 7, 2020, from www.nytimes.com/2020/07/07/nyregion/nyc-unemployment.html

The New York Times. (n.d.). Coronavirus in the U.S.: Latest map and case count. *The New York Times*. www.nytimes.com/interactive/2021/us/covid-cases.html
Oved, Y. (1988). *Two hundred years of American communes*. Transaction Books.
Pearson, D. (2023). *The ultimate prepper's Survival Bible*. Dale Pearson.
Pilon, M. (2016). *The monopolists*. Bloomsbury.
Schimmenti, A., Billieux, J., & Starcevic, V. (2020). The four horsemen of fear: An integrated model of understanding fear experiences during the COVID-19 pandemic. *Clinical Neuropsychiatry: Journal of Treatment Evaluation*, *17*(2), 41–45. https://psycnet.apa.org/record/2020-27302-001
Shepard, R. F. (1991, January 4). Halls of history, fame, oddity, and wonder. *The New York Times*. www.nytimes.com/1991/01/04/arts/halls-of-history-fame-oddity-and-wonder.html
Stewart, N., & Heisler, T. (2020). 1.5 million New Yorkers can't afford food. Pantries are their lifeline. *The New York Times*. www.nytimes.com/interactive/2020/10/20/nyregion/nyc-food-banks.html
United States Congress. (2017). *Joint economic committee*. www.jec.senate.gov/public/index.cfm/republicans/2017/2/2017-joint-economic-report
Waddell, N., Overall, N. C., & Hammond, M. D. (2021). Gendered division of labor during a nationwide COVID-19 lockdown: Implications for relationship problems and satisfaction. *Journal of Social and Personal Relationships*, *38*(6). https://doi.org/10.1177/0265407521996476
Williams, R. (1975). *The country and the city*. Oxford University Press.
Wright, K. (2022). *Community resilience: A critical approach*. Routledge.

6

FOSTERING RESILIENCE

The New York City Prepper's Network

The Last of Us, Season 1, Episode 3 – that's one. As someone who studies the prepper subculture, I have watched many American films and television shows to analyze depictions of preppers and the apocalypse. Preppers are frequently portrayed as eccentric, obsessed people who may just be seeking the end of the world because they are so alienated from their current existence. Preppers are never the heroes of the story. "I'm so glad that Steve has some duct tape and a tarp," said no one ever in one of these productions. Instead, prepper narratives usually focus on isolation and alienation. However, Episode 3 of The Last of Us broke away from the confines of such a narrative. It keeps me awake at night. It gets to the core of why many people seem to prepare for disaster. Through the story of a relationship between two men, the episode reveals that the practice of prepping is not merely skills development and stockpiling. Rather, the story suggests that, for some individuals, prepping might be grounded in a deeper understanding of purpose and community. As Murray (2023) explains, "over that 20-year stretch, we see the story of a love affair – doubling as a short, sweet lesson about what survival really means."

The Last of Us television series on HBO is actually based on a best-selling video game series of the same name. Released in 2013, the game has sold over 37 million copies (Carter, 2023). Both the TV show and the game are set in a world where a global pandemic has produced zombies and destroyed civilizations. A tough survivor, Joel, and a teenage girl, Ellie, undertake a dangerous journey across the country and depend on one another for survival. For Peter Hoar, the director of the series, the episode epitomizes the series' main theme: "'Life can be that tough, but what shines through is the humanity and the

DOI: 10.4324/9781003400356-6

hope. There has to be hope somewhere. You have to go looking for it, but it has to be there'" (Monteil, 2023; para. 11).

Departing from the central story of Joel and Ellie's struggles, Episode 3 is a flashback episode showing the events of the previous 20 years in the life of Bill (Nick Offerman), a friend of Joel's. Following the collapse of his small town during the pandemic, Bill, a seasoned prepper and now the town's only resident, springs into action. His prepping knowledge sustains him, and over time, he transforms the town into a fortress protected by traps and flamethrowers, which he commands from a high-tech bunker in his basement. Rather than subsisting on freeze-dried foods, he prepares elaborate meals of game that he has caught and vegetables that he has grown – not to mention the fine wine that he has stockpiled. Four years into Bill's story, Frank (Murray Bartlett), an uninfected traveler, is snared by one of Bill's traps. Convinced by Frank to let him survive and grateful for company, Bill makes a feast for lunch. Soon enough, the two fall in love (see Murray, 2023, for a beautiful summary).

As the years pass, Frank introduces an important new element of prepping to Bill – namely, trusting and building relationships for mutual support with other survivors such as Joel and his girlfriend. In one poignant scene, we discover that Frank has traded a handgun from Bill's arsenal for a pack of strawberry seeds – a resource for a pleasure. On Bill's birthday, Frank treats him to the delight of fresh strawberries. Unexpected sweetness in the apocalypse continues for some time until Frank develops a terminal illness. With Frank's health declining quickly, the two men enjoy one last good day together and drink wine mixed with too many painkillers before turning in. Bill explains to Frank that he is ready to pass: "You were my purpose. I am old. I am satisfied." Weeks later, Joel and Ellie arrive at the home of the couple. Bill has left a note for Joel that acknowledges that they are similar men and leaves the keys and codes for all of his provisions so that Joel may carry on with his own purpose of protecting those he loves.

Why are preppers almost never the heroes of the story? Why do we never thank Steve for always coming through with his duct tape? We tend to see preppers as isolated from the rest of us – not always in the literal sense of hiding in a bunker, although this certainly applies when we first meet Bill in a flashback to 2003. Rather, preppers are isolated in the sense that they seem so preoccupied with a world fallen apart, leaving behind the rest of us in the "normal" world and taking for granted the reality we have. Bill, however, shows us that this is anything but the case.

Many preppers were moved by the episode. For them, it emphasizes that knowledge, purpose, and connection are central to the philosophy of prepping. Jason was glad to see that a TV show depicted "a well-rounded prepper" engaging in tasks that, with the "right knowledge, someone could really do." While he was uncomfortable talking about a relationship between two men, he acknowledged that "the dynamics of the relationship" were very important to their success in surviving. In recommending the episode to me, Inshirah explained why she was so taken with it:

> It makes the right point. This isn't about going it alone. So what if you learn everything and you are there by yourself? What is the good in that? People need to be together to support one another, to trade, to learn things from one another. That's really the only way that this is going to work. It's about being together.

In the spirit of trying to figure out "how" and "why" being part of a community is so beneficial, this chapter explores prepping in New York City as an act of community resilience that seeks to strengthen preparedness and social networks as well as addressing the inequitable distribution of resources during disaster. Drawing from Hall and Lamont (2012, p. 232), community resilience refers to a social group's ability "to sustain its well-being in the face of challenges." Drivers of resilience are the experiences that group members hold in common as well as the organizational frameworks that form them. How does participation in a prepping group foster resiliency? By analyzing the process of how and the rationale behind why New Yorker preppers prepare for disasters, we can see how community members actually take on the task of learning resiliency. Their belief in self-reliance, approaches to survival (sheltering in place or leaving the city), gathering resources (supplies and skills), and networking are important factors that help the NYC Prepper's Network (NYCPN) members mobilize for action.

The NYCPN is not posited as a model for forming community resiliency groups. Instead, my purpose is to explore the activities of this group for what it is – an authentic local response to survival in a city of increased risk. In analyzing how NYCPN members prepared for and responded to the pandemic, this research reveals the power of community in mobilizing for and responding to disaster. It explores how a group conceptualizes its vulnerabilities and works to overcome these challenges independently of government direction or support. Therefore, the work of the NYCPN is examined according to two central components of community resilience: preparation and planning and response and recovery (Wright, 2022).

Preparation and planning refer to how individuals try to reduce their vulnerability to potential disaster through preventative actions like gaining knowledge about relevant risks, stockpiling basic provisions, preparing an emergency cache of tools and supplies (known as a bug-out bag to preppers), securing a safe haven, and creating an emergency plan (Paton et al., 2006; Rivera, 2020). Response refers to efforts to minimize the impact of the direct and indirect effects caused by disaster (Anderson, 2017). Recovery is more rooted in the work of government as it focuses on both the long-term efforts to rebuild and to help heal the physical and mental well-being of disaster victims. Determining a clear path for the city's recovery is explored in subsequent chapters of this book.

The rise of prepping in New York is not a phenomenon that can be analyzed solely according to the national political context. Rather, urban prepping is about adapting to the changing nature of life as a city dweller. It is about local, everyday choices, planning for the future, and thinking about community. As explained by one New York Times reader in the comments section about the impact of COVID-19 on New York: "Being a New Yorker takes work." What is the work of community resilience? Norris et al. (2007) argue the following:

> To build collective resilience, communities must reduce risk and resource inequities, engage local people in mitigation, create organizational linkages, boost and protect social supports, and plan for not having a plan, which requires flexibility, decision-making skills, and trusted sources of information that function in the face of unknowns.
>
> *(p. 127)*

To better understand urban prepping as a process for helping communities to plan and respond to disaster, this analysis draws on the framework of five capacities for community resilience (Faulkner et al., 2018): place attachment; leadership; knowledge and learning; community networks; and community cohesion and efficacy. Place attachment refers to the emotional, intellectual, and physical relationships that people have with place (Lewicka, 2001). It may bolster community resilience by motivating adaptation to maintain valued qualities of place (Amundsen, 2013) or undermine adaptation through resistance to new ideas and approaches (Marshall, 2007). Leadership is a process that encompasses individuals, organizations, roles, and actions that influence outcomes. The presence or absence of leadership impacts the development of critical components such as knowledge and trust building needed for resilience. Knowledge and learning refer to individual and group capacities to respond to local needs and issues (Maclean et al., 2014). These capacities involve learning new types of knowledge to improve the response to change (Magis, 2010) as well as learning from past crises to strengthen social memory (Wilson, 2012). Community networks involve the bonding and linking of ties that allow people to act collectively (Woolcock & Narayan, 2000). Establishing ties across diverse networks strengthens community resilience by opening up new outlets for support and resources as well as providing a renewed optimism during challenging times (Maclean et al., 2014).

Community cohesion and efficacy represent a community's ability to perform a task and manage prospective situations (Brown & Westaway, 2011). It centers on a community's sense of agency and its ability to develop its own level of resilience (Magis, 2010).

In the urban context, public education on disaster preparedness is made more complex by the diversity and distribution of vulnerable groups throughout a city (Paton & Johnston, 2001). Yet the NYCPN has successfully linked intention to action by fostering preparedness among its members (Dekens, 2007). Using Faulkner et al.'s (2018) framework to study the NYCPN is strategic because its categories of resilience capacities allow detailed analysis into the two types of social capital, bonding and bridging (Putnam, 2000), which work together to build resilience. Bonding social capital promotes cohesion, solidarity, and civic action (Mathbor, 2007). Bridging capital involves heterogeneous actors connecting across different networks to gain resources and achieve objectives (Consoer & Milman, 2016). For example, disaster planners and coordinators are traditionally responsible for transfers of human and material resources; however, the case of the NYCPN demonstrates how preppers create networks to provide support and resources for one another when government entities are unable to do so.

Place Attachment

Founded in 2010, NYCPN was created as a community of city dwellers dedicated to learning more about prepping. According to the NYCPN's Meetup page:

> The primary goal of the NYC Prepper's Network is to create a community network of like-minded individuals who share their knowledge of all things related to self-sufficiency . . . to establish a network of folks to share ideas with, learn from and eventually hope to trust should the need arise.
> *(2019)*

This mission statement reflects the NYCPN's core principles: learning from one another, demonstrating commitment by participating in training and excursions, and proving to be trustworthy. What meaning does New York have for these urban preppers in relation to planning for disaster? According to Tuan (1975, p. 156), cities are "central to meaning," not merely geographic locations. Rather, cities are social and cultural spaces that, through providing experiences and interactions, help define the character and aspirations of individuals. Place attachment can be seen as a dominant theme in the NYCPN's mission and conceptualization of prepping in three ways. First, before the pandemic, according to NCYPN members, New York's recent disaster history required that one should know how to prepare for survival. Second, once the pandemic reached the city, New York's position as the first epicenter of the pandemic in the context of the federal government's ambiguous plan for combatting the virus also worked to reinforce the group's philosophy of preparedness and self-reliance. Third, the confines of city life – a dense population living in smaller dwellings – require urban preppers to make adaptations to their survival strategies.

As the 21st century dawned, New York experienced disasters or threats of disasters of primary concern to urban preppers: terrorist attacks, technological failures, natural disasters, government or economic collapse, and pandemics. These direct experiences with disaster have driven interest in urban prepping. While the World Trade Center Attack of 2001 is well known, Manhattan also experienced four other terrorist attacks: the failed car bombing of Times Square in 2010; the Chelsea bomb explosion of 2016; a truck driven into people on the West Side bike path in 2017, and the partial detonation of a bomb in the Times Square-Port Authority subway in 2017. In 2012, New York was battered by Superstorm Sandy, the worst storm in the city's history. The 2003 Northeastern blackout also left New Yorkers without electricity for nearly two days, including thousands who were without mass transit. The Great Recession in 2008 also negatively affected the city's economy. As an international gateway, New York has always been in danger of the possible outbreak of pandemics or epidemics. While the city did not have significant outbreaks of Zika in 2016 or Ebola in 2014, New York endured an outbreak of H1N1 influenza (swine flu) in 2009.

For New York, as the first epicenter of COVID-19, and for the United States, the devastating impact of the pandemic across all areas of life – health, economic, and social – increased due to the federal government's failure to launch a comprehensive plan to battle the disease. Serious policy mistakes can be traced throughout the chronology of the virus's spread, including President Trump's decision to downplay early warnings about the virus, the government's failure to coordinate a national supply-chain for protective equipment and medical supplies, and the shifting policies on the wearing of facemasks (Shear et al., 2020). For New York preppers, the breakdown in governmental response at the federal level confirmed their belief in self-reliance. The pandemic had a more significant impact on the city than the 9/11 terrorist attack, the Great Recession, or Superstorm Sandy (Partnership for New York City, 2020). As President Trump continued to deny the effects of the pandemic, a weary city turned its eyes toward Governor Andrew Cuomo of New York State. Under Cuomo's direction, the New York State government and New York City government played tug-of-war while attempting to carry out a coordinated plan to address critical healthcare challenges such as bed shortages, overwhelmed hospital staff, and a lack of personal protective equipment for hospital workers.

With their suspicions of the government's failure during a crisis confirmed, many NYCPN members relied on their identities as New Yorkers and attachment to their city in becoming sources of strength and resilience in coping with living in the country's first epicenter of the virus. Place attachment encouraged many NYCPN members to shelter in place rather than leave. As Jason stated:

> I stayed because I'm a New Yorker. Sure, I get sick of the city sometimes, but it's my home. Some New Yorkers I know, they are real New Yorkers. They aren't going anywhere no matter what. There's only one New York. They are right about that.

Other NYCPN members also shared that their attachment to New York helped ground them when encountering negative responses about New York's need for aid during the height of the pandemic. Joseph, a four-year NYCPN member, explained:

> Reading Facebook comments like "New York can die" or "Let those liberal New Yorkers infect each other'" just disgusted me. New York's always rescuing other parts of the country. Every time there's a hurricane, we bail out some poor southern state. Still, they voted "no" on helping us after Hurricane Sandy. Remember, it took Jon Stewart to shame the country into helping 9/11 first-responders. New York preppers know that we can't depend on the feds or the states. Now, everyone else is starting to figure that out. I'm proud to be a New Yorker. New York's culture and money drive this country. We don't need them.
>
> The group's Meetup page also identifies the unique challenges of prepping in the city: NYC Preppers Network is an Emergency Preparedness & Wilderness group for city dwellers that are concerned with preparing for disasters. Some of us don't live in a home, have garages, wells, basements, or attics to store our survival gear in. Most of us live in apartments. City occupants face a different set of challenges. Space, Food Storage, Water, Security, Sanitation, Evacuation Routes & many other issues are of a great concern for city dwellers. (NYCPN, 2019)

In describing the challenges of prepping in New York, which include limited space for storing supplies and few evacuation routes, the group also connects to the emotional, intellectual, and physical relationships to place. High population density, traffic congestion and smaller dwellings are all challenges of New York life that make prepping even more difficult. For urban preppers, the two main approaches to surviving disaster are sheltering in place ("bugging in") and leaving the city to reach a safe haven ("bugging out"). In these two approaches, the social and physical dimensions of place attachments can work to promote or weaken resilience.

Bugging out refers to leaving an area to escape disaster. In planning for bugging out of the city, the city's physical characteristics such its geography, travel routes, and exit points are foregrounded over its social dimensions.

When using this strategy, New York preppers plan to leave the city for safe havens, which can include the home of a family member or friend, a second home, or a hidden campsite in the tri-state area. New York preppers would rely on their own bug-out bags for food and supplies until they reach their safe destination. Given traffic congestion and the limited number of exit routes, leaving the city by car or bus may prove difficult. With advance warning, some NYCPN members planned to drive or fly out of the city. For example, some NYCPN members elected to leave the city in response to early warnings about the high risks of COVID-19 to city residents.

Leadership

The existence of NYCPN, a public group for preppers, runs counter to traditional notions about the prepping subculture. Preppers are thought to be secretive about their level of preparedness (their supplies) for two reasons. First, they are concerned about being stigmatized as crazy, paranoid people who are suspicious of everyone, especially the government. Second, they are also concerned about being identified as preppers because, in the event of a disaster, they fear that they will be attacked because they have provisions. According to Jason Charles, the leader of NYCPN, there is some truth to both of these assertions. He argues that most preppers are not crazy or paranoid. Instead, they are people who understand, usually from direct experience, that the world is becoming a riskier place. However, they are suspicious of government because it continues to fail its citizens. Some preppers are also concerned about being discovered because they are fearful of an attack. Jason believes that they could certainly be attacked in a SHFT (Shit Hits the Fan) situation; therefore, preppers should plan to protect themselves. Yet Jason continues to be a spokesperson for prepping. When I asked him about the threat of such an attack, he shrugged his shoulders and said, "Yeah, I've thought about it. The neighbors see the cameras [the media] and everything. I'm more interested in making sure that people understand why and how to prep. That's what matters." Of course, Jason's linebacker physique and his knife skills probably matter, too.

In 2012, America first met Jason, the urban prepper, on National Geographic's record-breaking television series Doomsday Preppers in an episode titled "Escape from New York." Slinging a giant tree over his shoulder like a flimsy D'Agostino's bag, Jason captivated viewers with his rugged good looks, powerful body, and straightforward style.[1] Despite the show's sensationalism and mockery of its informants (Genzlinger, 2012), the episode revealed that prepping was not a practice reserved for the stereotype of rural White men who were suspicious of government and people unlike them. Through Jason's appearance, viewers discovered that prepping transcended geography, class, and race. As an African-American male living in New York City, Jason presents a very surprising image that reflects the diversity of preppers. His appearance revealed to viewers that preppers can also be city dwellers and people of color. He's in newspapers, he's on TV, he's on social media, he's on YouTube, he's on podcasts, and he leads NYCPN meetings. Googling "Jason Charles, Prepper" now results in nearly 700,000 hits. There is no denying his identity as a prepper. His is the face of New York City prepping.

Jason has spent most of his life helping people deal with emergencies. Now retired, Jason served in the New York Fire Department for over 20 years, and he has been a prepper for 12 years. He has guided the NYCPN's mission and activities since 2012. His dedication to teaching preparedness is rooted in his experience as a first responder and in his survivalist training. In addition to earning numerous certifications, he has completed two rigorous Wilderness Survival training programs, The Pathfinder School in Ohio and The Mountain Scout Survival School in New York. This training reinforced his belief that survival success is rooted in experiential learning rather than merely discussing prepping strategies. After mastering new skills, Jason then teaches them to the group. In addition, Jason improves and shares his prepping knowledge by reviewing new gear and testing out equipment innovations. During his tenure, the group's focus has shifted from only holding meetings to practicing survival skills during organized outdoor excursions.

In making the critical shift from discussion to action, leadership was practiced as a process, not as a position (Curphy et al., 1999). While Charles was the primary leader, co-organizers assisted him in implementing the group's new agenda and activities. Co-organizers are selected based on their seniority in the group, commitment to participation, and their respective skills sets. Their role was broad and included teaching and administrative tasks such as designing and leading workshops, planning events, screening for membership, and scouting locations for excursions.

In 2020, the NYCPN had a diverse roster of nearly 500 members.[2] The majority of group members were people of color, including African Americans, Afro-Caribbean, Puerto Ricans, and Asians. NYCPN members reside in all five boroughs with most members living in Manhattan, the Bronx, Queens, and Brooklyn. Some members also now live in New Jersey, but they still participate in the group. NYCPN members vary in age, from early twenties to senior citizens. Members also hold jobs in diverse economic sectors such as emergency response, law, security, technology, tourism, business-to-business, and education.

Wright (2022, p. 77) argues that "the preppers' highly individualist approach to resilience can seem to involve a withdrawal and disaffiliation from social obligations. . . . This seems antithetical to – and potentially undermines – ideals of community resilience and shared social security." However, NYCPN's purpose and organizational leadership actually seem to provide a foundation for bolstering community resilience.

Knowledge and Learning

Gaining knowledge and skills is the primary focus of the NYCPN. To facilitate learning disaster preparedness, NYCPN engages in activities ranging from lectures to weekend excursions at various skill levels. Members are expected to demonstrate a deep commitment to prepping through active participation and developing advanced bushcraft skills and sheltering-in-place capabilities. During its 13-year history, the NYCPN has held over 100 meetings. Meeting types include general meetings and topic discussions, lectures and workshops where members learn a new skill, attending events not sponsored by the group but related to prepping, and excursions, including two-day retreats and overnight outings to practice skills. The group's agenda has advanced from exploring introductory topics to focusing on practicing prepping skills in outdoor settings. For the first three years, 2010–2012, the group's activities centered on developing basic prepping and homesteading knowledge such as learning the purpose and contents of a bug-out bag and an introduction to canning through lectures, workshops, and events. Starting in 2013, the group's agenda expanded to include excursions like challenging bug-out trips and hands-on workshops on more advanced homesteading skills such as making leather crafts and toiletries. From 2014 through 2019, overnight excursions to practice skills and to develop endurance were the group's top activity. Before the pandemic, this level of training provided members with not just skills but also with increased confidence in their ability to deal with disaster. In 2020, the majority of the meetings were virtual. In 2021–2022, excursions once again became the group's top activity. As one NYCPN member of three years observed:

> Training with the group was crucial to my knowing how to deal with the pandemic. Our trips have toughened me up a bit. I wasn't anxious. I was steady and trying to figure the best plan for my family. Being part of the NYCPN, I had protective gear and my stores. We learned how to shelter in place. The real lesson for me, what I learned from the group, was breaking down my plan into components that made sense for a pandemic, making adjustments for the long haul, not just a few days and making sure we had some flexibility. Feeling confident about my choices.

In the weeks before the COVID-19 pandemic struck the city, NYCPN members were already prepared to shelter in place, with their prepper closets stocked with provisions required during a pandemic, such as personal protective equipment. Given the shortage of hand sanitizer and its spike in pricing, Jason taught a workshop on how to make hand sanitizer. Inshirah, a senior member who specialized in homesteading, also offered a workshop on food dehydration and canning to ensure that members had access to vegetables and fruits in the event of shortages. Once the outbreak occurred, the NYCPN responded by holding virtual meetings that addressed issues related to coping with COVID-19 and to exchange ideas and tips for making sheltering in place in the city easier for city dwellers.

It is also important to note that the NYCPN meetings were open to the public, so all interested individuals could attend. Through these events, NYCPN members and other attendees learned different types and forms of knowledge that allow them to respond and adapt to change (MacLean et al., 2014). Topics were varied. Open discussions were held about New York being the epicenter of the pandemic and frustrations over the lack of concern in other parts of the country. Sheltering-in-place discussions were also held that encouraged preppers to stay the course and to make adjustments for quarantining in small spaces such as adhering to a schedule and designating work and study spaces. Members also exchanged information about identifying areas that now appeared to be less safe due to the pandemic, as well as identifying local stores that carried needed supplies and seemed to restock quickly. In speaking about the group's importance to her during lockdown, Inshirah stated:

> The group has helped me have a sense of appreciation for people who think ahead. During the pandemic, I had a few moments of wondering how I would do if things get much worse. Having people to rely on is crucial.

Still, there was some disagreement during meetings. Prior to the pandemic, the NYCPN banned any discussion of politics. However, as political battles became central to the government's efforts to manage the pandemic, the ban was lifted. A few members who had joined at the start of the pandemic disagreed with political viewpoints presented by Jason during online meetings. After Jason complained about China's reluctance to share information, a Chinese prepper voiced her concern about singling out China as a bad actor and that such comments might lead to an increase in hate crimes against Asian Americans. Jason accepted her comment, but he did not retract his remarks. In an April meeting, a new member sent me a note that read, "He only wants to talk about his opinion. He doesn't care about what I have to say." I did not recognize the person's name, and I received no response to my reply. (The person had the camera turned off). In the chat, I then discovered that a few new members had started using an encrypted messaging app for private conversations. As a researcher, I was curious to see if the encrypted conversation would lead to an outcome like a closed network within the group or possibly produce an offshoot of the group. However, the encrypted messaging subgroup quickly disbanded. It was spearheaded by a new member, an older male, who seemed to be interested in using the encrypted messaging app to talk with female members and to try to persuade them of his suitability as the new leader of the group. His interest in talking only with women and trying to convince them to continue sharing encrypted messages was viewed as disturbing by two of the female members that he had contacted. Based on discussions with the women, Inshirah determined that his behavior represented a creepy overture rather an attempt at trying to become the group's leader. Information sharing among female group members also revealed that his actions were similar in a different (non-prepping) group, and he was subsequently removed from the NYCPN.

Community Cohesion

The NYCPN benefits from strong community cohesion. Central to community cohesion are agency and self-efficacy – key attributes that enable communities to plan, manage, and adapt to disaster (Brown & Westwood, 2011). Agency is the capacity of a group to engage independently in collective action to define its own resilience. Self-efficacy is the community's collective belief in its capacity to perform behaviors necessary to meet their objective. In other words, community cohesion hinges on the independence and will of the group. Through their training and real-life application of prepping skills during COVID-19, the members of the NYCPN have demonstrated their collective ability to endure disaster. Their commitment to self-reliance and their belief in their prepping skills have empowered them to protect their families and neighbors during a crisis. Their resilience is founded on their commitment to and trust in one another.

In studying emergent response groups, Majchrzak et al. (2007, p. 159) found that in dangerous settings, trust stems from "purposive action that conveys investment and vulnerability." In the emotional and physical strain of disasters, trust is dynamic and continuously reaffirmed through action. Trust as a dynamic and continuous force (Adler, 2001) is a core value of the NYCPN because it is a central component of preparedness. Trustworthiness is first measured by a group member's dedication to learning survival skills by participating in NYCPN activities. During challenging outdoor excursions, known as "bug outs," NYCPN members bond with one another through overcoming hardships as the group works collectively to survive by completing tasks such as fire making, shelter building, or finding a water source. In a disaster, performing fundamental survival skills and knowing how to use one's tools enable a prepper to respond and adapt to a situation more quickly. Rather than struggling with how to build a fire for the first time, for example, a well-prepared prepper in a disaster will be able to focus efforts on other matters such as building a shelter or aiding other survivors. Most important, bug-out trips expose preppers to the experience of adapting to the stress of surviving in a difficult, unfamiliar scenario.

Prior to the pandemic, a bug-out bag symbolized a prepper's level of trustworthiness and competence level in a survival situation. Typically weighing around 20 pounds, a bug-out bag is a pre-packed bag with emergency essentials for at least a five-day period (Charles, 2014). It contains crucial provisions such as water, food, first aid, shelter, clothing, fire, tools, and reference documents (see www.ready.gov/build-a-kit for a supply list). Beyond must-have items, many supplies are selected according to personal preference. NYCPN members create bags for themselves by carefully selecting and testing their own provisions to ensure optimal quality and durability. On excursions, members rely on the contents of their respective bug-out bags for survival. Therefore, a member's knowledge of and familiarity with one's tools is an important indicator of a person's commitment to prepping. It is also an invaluable indicator of honesty. Someone may tell you that she or he is a seasoned prepper and may even recount a clever story or two that showcases her or his abilities. However, the real truth is hidden in the bug-out bag. If the bag's tools and supplies are new and untested, so is the prepper. Seasoned preppers test and practice with their equipment.

As the pandemic continued, a prepper's closet became an important symbol of trustworthiness. The careful stocking and maintenance of provisions is a complex process that offers great insight into one's knowledge about sheltering in place. Group members already had protective equipment and food stored for potential use; therefore, they frequently discussed their provisions and compared notes on cost, quality, and shelf life. Furthermore, NYCPN members exchanged information about strategies for extending the shelf life of food items, expanding the number of servings of freeze-dried provisions and creative storage options for small apartments (such as utilizing storage underneath beds or in bookcases). These discussions strengthen the knowledge base of and the bond between group members, and these conversations also allow members to demonstrate their competence and commitment to the group, elevating their status. Given the shortage of masks and the requirement to wear a mask in public places, members would sometimes discuss new types of masks (supposedly similar to N-95 masks), critiquing and evaluating their quality and safety. For example, the group once discussed the new type of clear face shield with a HEPA filter that was being lauded as better than an N-95 mask, with the benefit of being able to show your entire face. This face shield was being launched on Kickstarter. The group's discussion of the new face shield revealed flaws in the construction of the mask that would permit the transmission of the airborne virus. I regret that I should have probably talked with these preppers before ordering the face shields (which were never delivered because the company went bankrupt).

The creation of a satisfactory bug-out bag and prepper's closet are important achievements for NYCPN members. Rather than merely being items, the bug-out bag and the prepper closet each represent a survival approach that can be carried out through the use of knowledge and tools. The NYCPN provides strong bonding capital because these two survival approaches improve the resiliency of NYCPN members. Through their participation in the NYCPN, members have gained valuable resources to protect their families against disaster without relying on government aid or action. This level of resilience is crucial for vulnerable and marginalized people who have experienced inequities in the distribution of aid during disaster, not only because they usually live in neighborhoods that are more exposed but also because they lack the resources needed for coping with the aftermath (Wisner et al., 2003), which negatively impacts recovery outcomes (Phillips & Fordham, 2010).

Community Networks

Through its events and the existing connections of group members, the NYCPN also strengthens its resilience by fostering links to diverse networks. As a group, the NYCPN establishes connections with experts in preparedness and organizations that teach survival skills. Before the pandemic, the NYCPN invited guest speakers to share their insights at meetings, where group leaders convey information about organizations and resources. NYCPN members also attend training or events and report back to the group about their respective experiences. This ongoing exchange of information and resources (such as innovations in prepping skills or equipment) strengthens group resilience and their sense of community.

Although preppers are sometimes stereotyped by the media as paranoid isolationists, NYCPN members have strong social networks, and many belong to civic organizations. Work-based networks are also critical, as some NYCPN members are employed in the emergency services, healthcare, and public services. Through these networks, the NYCPN is able to receive and exchange timely and valuable information regarding disasters. By participating in civic organizations and other volunteer groups, NYCPN members utilized social networks as information and resource links throughout the pandemic.

In late January 2020, as concerns about the COVID-19 pandemic began to grow, many NYCPN members started to exchange ideas about the potential threat of the pandemic and to discuss their respective approaches to sheltering in place. In the weeks before the pandemic, many urban preppers, secure in their own preparations, began to teach their neighbors and friends how to shelter in place. By replying to texts, answering phone calls, and coaching people on purchases, NYCPN members worked as trusted advisors in disaster preparedness. As one urban prepper observed, "For years, no one wanted to talk with me about prepping. I was a crazy person. Now, everyone is calling me for advice. That's fine. I'm happy to help. At last." The willingness of

NYC preppers to give advice about preparing for the pandemic was possibly an important contribution to community preparedness. Rivera (2020) found that the likelihood of someone developing a household emergency plan increased with previous exposure to disaster and to preparedness information.

During the COVID-19 pandemic, NYCPN members benefited from the mutual assistance offered by mobilizing these networks. Information was exchanged regarding breaking news about government policies on protecting against the virus and advice from city healthcare workers. For example, some NYCPN members are first responders who provided updates on neighborhoods hit especially hard by the pandemic, overcrowded hospitals, or areas with increasing crime rates. Interstate and intrastate resource networks that allowed for the distribution of needed supplies also emerged. Through these networks, calls were made for supplies so that others could try to locate the items, and supplies were either exchanged between members, offered for free, or sold for face value. In one network of restaurant suppliers and friends, NYCPN members were kept abreast of the availability of highly sought food items such as yeast and flour. In another network, one New York prepper opened up her large cache of provisions to non-preppers in need. Lastly, after several family members contracted COVIV-19 due to employment that required face-to-face interaction, Hassan relied on a network of medical supplies to secure Ivermectin tablets for all six people. Similar to Consoer and Milman's (2016) study of the role of social capital of recovery groups in Vermont after Tropical Storm Irene, the NYCPN's successful web of community networks illustrates that strong bonding social capital attracted bridging social capital, which allowed access to more available resources.

As an example of community resilience, the NYCPN demonstrates how human interaction, resources, and social capital can bolster a group's success in contending with disaster (Chaskin, 2008). Exploring the mission and activities of the NYCPN according to Faulkner et al.'s (2018) framework of five capacities for community resilience revealed the importance of each element and their interconnections in shaping the resilience of a community. For these urban preppers, place attachment served as a foundation for building their group's agenda and their respective survival plans. Analyzing the social and physical dimensions of New York as a place for survival or a place to escape from was central to all levels of preparedness. The NYCPN's goals of teaching and practicing survival skills on excursions required leadership in many forms. While the group's primary leader served as both a spokesperson and educator, as an individual he could not complete all the management tasks without the support of dedicated members. Given the NYCPN's mission to acquire preparedness skills, knowledge and learning were core principles of the group. Community cohesion was reinforced throughout preparedness training as group members learned to develop their individual skills and to rely on one another. The creation of a bug-out bag and a prepper's closet are two valuable resources for resiliency gained by participating in the group. The NYCPN's diverse networks also enabled members to assist one another as well as nongroup members.

The NYCPN's mission and activities demonstrate possible ways to engage in the work of community resilience. Lacking a clear federal plan to combat the virus, the NYCPN sought to improve community resilience by educating New Yorkers about preparedness for disaster and, in response to disaster, developing networks to aid preppers and others. The group's work also points to the need to develop disaster management approaches that can expand the traditional "command and control" models to incorporating community-based involvement in disaster preparedness (LaLone, 2012). Making space for local knowledge and resources can only help to increase community resilience. By adopting this approach, disaster management professionals can build on a community's existing strengths.

Notes

1 At the start of Jason's segment, I am pretty sure that the music sounded something like "See me ride out of the sunset/On your color TV screen . . . I'm TNT." I could be wrong.
2 In 2023, the number of NYCPN members is 603.

References

Adler, P. S. (2001). Market, hierarchy, and trust: The knowledge economy and the future of capitalism. *Organization Science*, *12*(2), 215–234.

Amundsen, H. (2013). Place attachment as a driver of adaptation in coastal communities in Northern Norway. *Local Environment: The International Journal of Justice and Sustainability*, *20*(3), 237–276.

Anderson, B. (2017). Emergency futures: Exception, urgency, interval, hope. *The Sociological Review*, *65*(3), 463–477.

Brown, K., & Westaway, E. (2011). Agency, capacity, and resilience to environmental change: Lessons from human development, well-being, and disasters. *Annual Review of Environment and Resources*, *36*, 321–342. http://doi.org/10.1146/annurev-environ-052610-092905

Carter, J. (2023, January 4). The last of us franchise has sold 37 million copies in 9 years. *Game Developer*. www.gamedeveloper.com/business/the-last-of-us-franchise-has-sold-37-million-copies-in-9-years

Charles, J. (2014). *Emergency bag essentials: Everything you need to bug out*. Potter Style.

Chaskin, R. (2008). Resilience, community, and resilient communities: Conditioning contexts and collective action. *Child Care in Practice: Building Resilience in Children, Families and Communities*, *14*(1), 65–74.

Consoer, M., & Milman, A. (2016). The dynamic process of social capital during recovery from Tropical Storm Irene in Vermont. *Natural Hazards: Journal of the International Society for the Prevention and Mitigation of Natural Hazards*, *84*(1), 155–174.

Curphy, G. J., Ginnett, R. C., & Hughes, R. L. (1999). *Leadership: Enhancing the lessons of experience*. Irwin/McGraw Hill.

Dekens, J. (2007). *Local knowledge for disaster preparedness: A literature review*. International Centre for Integrated Mountain Development (ICIMOD).

Faulkner, L., Brown, K., & Quinn, T. (2018). Analyzing community resilience as an emergent property of dynamic social-ecological systems. *Ecology and Society*, *23*(1), 24.

Genzlinger, N. (2012, December 16). Dubious ideas, and hybrids that got away. *The New York Times*. www.nytimes.com/2012/12/16/arts/television/neil-genzlinger-on-tvs-missed-opportunities-in-2012.html

Hall, A., & Lamont, M. (2012). *Social resistance is the neo-liberal era*. Cambridge University Press.

LaLone, M. B. (2012). Neighbors helping neighbors: An examination of the social capital mobilization process for community resilience to environmental disasters. *Journal of Applied Social Science*, *6*(2), 209–237.

Lewicka, M. (2001). Place attachment: How far have we come in the last 40 years? *Journal of Environmental Psychology*, *31*(3), 207–230.

Maclean, K., Cuthill, M., & Ross, H. (2014). Six attributes of social resilience. *Journal of Environmental Planning and Management*, *54*(1), 144–156.

Magis, K. (2010). Community resilience: An indicator of social sustainability. *Society and Natural Resources*, *23*, 401–416.

Majchrzak, A., Jarvenpaa, S., & Hollingshead, A. (2007). Coordinating expertise among emergent groups responding to disasters. *Organization Science*, *18*(1), 147–161.

Marshall, N. A. (2007). Can policy perception influence social resilience to policy change? *Fisheries Research*, *86*, 216–227.

Mathbor, G. M. (2007). Enhancement of community preparedness for natural disasters: The role of social work in building social capital for sustainable disaster relief and management. *International Social Work*, *50*, 357–369.

Monteil, A. (2023, January 29). The last of us tells a hauntingly beautiful story of gay survival in its third episode. *Them*. www.them.us/story/the-last-of-us-episode-three-gay-love-story-peter-hoar-interview

Murray, N. (2023, January 29). "The last of us" season 1, episode 3 recap: One more good day. *The New York Times*. www.nytimes.com/2023/01/29/arts/television/the-last-of-us-recap-episode-3.html

New York City Prepper's Network (APN Chapter) (New York, NY). (2019). www.meetup.com/NYC-Preppers-Network/

Norris, F., Stevens, S. P., Pfefferbaum, B., Wyche, K., & Pfferbaum, R. L. (2007). Community resilience as a metaphor, theory, set of capacities, and strategy for disaster readiness. *American Journal of Community Psychology*, *41*, 127–150.

Paton, D., & Johnston, D. (2001). Disasters and communities: Vulnerability, resilience and preparedness. *Disaster Prevention and Management*, *10*(4), 270–277. https://doi.org/10.1108/EUM0000

Paton, D., McClure, J., & Burgelt, P. (2006). Natural hazard resilience: The role of individual and household preparedness. In D. Paton & D. Johnston (Eds.), *Disaster resilience: An integrated approach* (pp. 121–139). Charles C Thomas Publisher.

Phillips, B. D., & Fordham, M. (2010). Introduction. In B. D. Phillips, D. S. K. Thomas, A. Fothergill, & L. Blinn-Pike (Eds.), *Social vulnerability to disasters* (pp. 1–26). CRC Press.

Putnam, R. D. (2000). *Bowling alone: The collapse and revival of American community*. Simon & Schuster.

Rivera, J. (2020). The likelihood of having a household emergency plan: Understanding factors in the US context. *Natural Hazards (Dordrecht)*, *104*(2), 1331–1343.

Shear, M. D., Weiland, N., Lipton, E., Haberman, M., & Sanger, D. E. (2020, July 28). *Inside Trump's failure: The rush to abandon leadership role on the virus*. www.

nytimes.com/2020/07/18/us/politics/trump-coronavirus-response-failure-leadership.html
Tuan, Y. (1975). Place: An experiential perspective. *Geographical Review*, *65*(2), 151–165.
Wilson, G. A. (2012). *Community resilience and environmental transitions*. Routledge.
Wisner, B., Blaikie, P., Cannon, T., & Davis, I. (2003). *At risk: Natural hazards, people's vulnerability and disasters* (2nd ed.). Routledge.
Woolcock, M., & Narayan, D. (2000). Social capital: Implications for development theory, research, and policy. *World Bank Research Observer*, *15*(2), 25–49.
Wright, K. (2022). *Community resilience: A critical approach*. Routledge.

7

PREPPER ADVICE FOR POST-PANDEMIC NEW YORK

Like many New Yorkers, I gauge the city's mood according to my subway ride. When a homeless man harassed my friend from out of town for our entire ride from Union Square to Times Square, the city was feeling righteous: she had been making fun of homeless people all afternoon. These days, my subway rides tell me that the city is often anxious.

I didn't see them enter the car, but I could hear them. I was engaged in a staring contest with the British tourist seated across from me. He kept watching me like I was a New Yorker in the wild, so I stared at him blankly, but it backfired. Suddenly, we were locked in a no-blinking staring contest.

"Mind your own business!" Shouted the first woman.

"I saw what you did and it is a crime!" Yelled the second woman.

"I said 'mind your own fucking business'."

"I *am* minding my own business. I'm a New Yorker. This *is* my business."

To suggest that we might want to take a look, the Brit arched an eyebrow. I shrugged a shoulder and broke the gaze. I expected to see a teen girl and an older woman providing guidance to the younger female. Instead, I saw two professionally dressed women of roughly the same age. I turned back to the Brit. This time, he shrugged both shoulders. As their shouting continued, it became clear that one of the women had entered without paying.

"Didn't you see me? I was on the phone explaining that I'm late." (Actually, the fare skipper said a few more colorful things that I am too embarrassed to type.)

"It's a crime. We all can't just do whatever the hell we want now. It's a crime. This craziness has to stop!" The angry citizen, too, said a few more colorful things.

DOI: 10.4324/9781003400356-7

Wearing their nearly identical black wool dress coats with their fancy scarves, the women continued to argue as I got off the train. The Brit stayed on the train. He kept fiddling with his camera, eager to take a photo of the face-off.

The second woman's words stuck with me. It was clear that she wasn't just angry about the other person's decision to sneak in without paying. By yelling "all the craziness has to stop," she seemed to be angry about her perception that the city was no longer safe. Her comments reflected the mood of the city that day. Anxious. Angry. Fed up. At that time (November 2022), I hoped that this mood might pass and that our collective sensibility would transition back into something more closely resembling the city-dweller attitude of tolerance and indifference.[1] However, it is now summer 2023, and we have yet to make that return because, the truth is, many of us are still fearful and, well . . . things are all still a little unsettled. A recent Facebook post on "Into the Unknown," a page created during the pandemic for those contemplating leaving the city, expresses the overwhelming concerns that many now have about city life. In a 2023 conversation about the pros and cons of living in the city, one New Yorker commented:

> We're paying an absolutely absurd and unsustainable premium to stay in a neighborhood (been here 10+yrs) with a relatively low crime rate and both crime + unpleasant societal run-ins have increased in the past few years. I keep thinking that it's just my luck or that I'm getting old . . . but then I witness an assault or someone taking a sh*t in the street. Don't get me wrong, I've seen my fair share living in the city pre-pandemic, but now it seems constant . . . everywhere. Literally clawing my way to stay hoping things will improve, but edging on the admission that I'm living in denial. The reality is that cost of living keeps increasing and societal standards are decreasing. There no longer seems to be a somewhat balanced trade-off for bleeding funds to live here.

During the pandemic, most of our fears were closely tied to the immediate dangers of COVID-19. Schimmenti et al. (2020) argue that during the pandemic people experienced four interrelated domains of fear: (1) fear of the body/fear for the body, (2) fear of significant others/fear for significant others, (3) fear of not knowing/fear of knowing, and (4) fear of taking action/fear of inaction. Fear of the body involves physical vulnerability and alarm about the possible dangers of becoming infected. Fear for the body refers to valuing the body and seeking to protect it from harm. Fear of significant others stems from the recognition that close contact with our loved ones may harm us, whereas fear for our significant others involves changing our behaviors to better protect our loved ones from ourselves as a potential threat. To overcome the fear of not knowing (and the consequences of not knowing), securing any information about COVID-19 may have provided a sense of control or understanding. However, for some who experienced the fear of knowing, information about the real threat of COVID-19 could be overwhelming, making one feel vulnerable.

Now that the pandemic has ended, the long-term problems caused by COVID have moved to the forefront. New Yorkers are now fearful about issues such as the rise in crime (even though crime rate is not very high), an increase in mental health problems, an increase in homelessness, and the challenges to the city's economic recovery. As one Harlem resident explained to me:

> When it comes to thinking about all that we have been through as a city during the pandemic, we aren't using the word that we should be using. It is called "trauma." We haven't dealt with it. Now, we are all walking around with PTSD, trying to deal with all the new stuff.

The "new stuff?" Examples of new stressors include the city becoming a "Heat Island,"[2] the influx of poor migrants who deserve aid, and the poor air quality caused by the Canadian wildfires.[3] The sky was orange, remember? Who can forget it? Orange.

The anxiety about New York's current challenges is a reminder that all pandemics cause not only death and depopulation but also social and economic upheavals (Gordon, 2020). Moving on is not necessarily moving forward. Although three years have passed since lockdown, the rates of depression and anxiety among New Yorkers remain high. According to the New York Health Foundation (2023), 31.5% of New Yorkers experienced one or both conditions in 2023; this rate shows no improvement since 2021, when 32% of New Yorkers reported poor mental health. Furthermore, mental health issues were more common among people of color, young people, the poor, and the unemployed.

This chapter draws from the philosophy of prepping to offer an alternative perspective for analyzing New York's recovery and the city's future. The pandemic has demonstrated that practicing emergency preparedness was useful and that it was risky to rely only on aid from the government during a crisis. As Ryan (2015) notes, resilience is best derived from "top down" approaches as well as "bottom up" strategies and ordinary tactics. Therefore, this chapter explores a list of prepper adages to consider in planning for New York's future. Urban preppers can teach us much about the benefits of self-reliance – networking and community-building in a period of crisis. While their distrust in government is now commonplace among Americans, their practices are also potent reminders of the kind of power that an engaged citizenry can hold. Urban resilience demands both a strong city government and an engaged citizenry.

Practice Situational Awareness. For preppers, survival hinges on protection from physical and economic dangers, and, when disaster does strike, accurate assessments must be made of one's plight and future possibilities. Situational awareness is key and involves evaluating your surroundings for dangerous situations and potential threats to your safety (survivalistprepper.net, 2023). By analyzing your vulnerabilities and recognizing normal conditions (a baseline), the goal is to develop a plan of action for responding to or avoiding dangerous situations. This knowledge provides a certain level of control by being able to form expectations and possible responses. Similarly, to preppers, New Yorkers might consider examining the state of the city from a perspective of situational awareness. In thinking about post-pandemic New York, what sectors are now still so far from the baseline of their pre-pandemic levels that they should be viewed as threats to the city's vitality and economy? As Bhat and Welch (2023) explain:

> There is no one way of knowing how long it will take New York City to regain its pre-COVID mojo. When it comes to a pandemic that left New Yorkers emotionally traumatized and financially strained, the city's recovery is multifaceted, coming in fits and starts as new variants [and new problems] reverse or slow its momentum.

Analyzing the state of the city from a prepper's understanding of situational awareness discloses interesting tension. As outlined below, the state of the city is improving. Crime is falling and still historically low. The economy is in many ways healthy. Therefore, the main challenge might be that perception is the problem. Time is required to progress from "recovering" to "recovered." This might be one of the few times that New York has not provided immediate gratification for its residents.

Crime

Since the pandemic, fears about increased crime in the city have unnerved residents and visitors alike, perhaps especially those residents who have always been resistant to commuting. However, the perception of crime might have overpowered the reality of the city's safety (Akinnibi & Wahid, 2022). Crime increased in the city during the pandemic after reaching historic lows in the three previous years. Between 2017 and 2019, the New York Police Department (NYPD) reported fewer than 100,000 major crimes and fewer than 320 murders in each of the three years preceding the pandemic (NYPD, 2023). The city's murder rate was at its lowest level in decades just prior to the pandemic. To provide historical context, the city's crime rate increased year over year during the pandemic; however, the crime rate still remained lower than 2000 when Mayor Rudolf Guiliani held office (Pozarycki, 2022). During the 1980s and early 1990s, the murder rate was also five times higher than now with an average of six killings per day (Akinnibi & Wahid, 2022). Consider the 2022 murder rate (414 killings). From 2019 to 2022, the murder rate increased by 28.9% (from 319 to 414 killings). Yet in comparison to 1990, the year of the highest number of murders on record for the city (2,264 killings), the 2022 murder rate shows an 81.6% decrease with 1,834 fewer killings.[4] The 2023 rate, year-to-date, remains below 2022, with homicides decreasing by 10% (269 versus 298) in comparison to the previous year's first eight months (NYPD, 2023).

Our collective sense of fear may also be linked to increased media attention as some of the recent homicides have occurred in public spaces.[5] Violent crimes in subway stations and in tourist areas have fueled anxiety that crime has significantly increased. Unfortunately, examples are numerous. On a Saturday morning, a woman was shoved in front of a moving train at the Times Square station (Closson & Newman, 2022). On a crowded subway car headed from Brooklyn to Manhattan, a man set off smoke grenades and then opened fire, injuring 23 people – 10 by gunfire. (Nir & Newman, 2022). In Lower Manhattan, a man on his way to brunch was fatally shot in a subway car in an unprovoked attack (Southall & Schweber, 2022). The horrific nature of these violent events has shaken the confidence of New Yorkers. For example, a Quinnipiac University poll (2022) found that 49% of registered voters felt that crime was the most urgent issue facing New York now. Also, 86% of these voters supported having more police officers in the subway system. The perception of a lack of safety in the city has also been influenced by Mayor Adams's "tough on crime" rhetoric during both his campaign and his administration.

Homelessness

In June 2023, New York sadly set a new record of over 100,000 people in the city's homeless shelter system (the majority being families with children) (Newman, 2023). Beginning in spring 2022, the city's shelter system has been overwhelmed with a massive influx of migrants from the nation's southern border. The number of nonmigrants in the city's shelter system is also growing, currently numbering 50,000. The city government has appealed to the federal and state governments for assistance in providing aid to migrants. The city government has already spent $1 billion in providing shelter and support to this program, and Mayor Adams plans to spend $4 billion in the next year (Newman, 2023). With no more indoor space available, Adams has indicated that outdoor alternatives will now be employed, such as tents in certain sections of the city (Fitzsimmons & Root, 2023). Compare these figures to 2019 when the city provided shelter to 63,839 people nightly (Routhier, 2019).

Subway Ridership

At the start of the pandemic, subway ridership fell by over 90% (Bhat & Welch, 2023). While it has improved, subway ridership remains significantly lower than 2019 levels. In February 2023, subway ridership was at 65% of pre-pandemic levels (up from 56% at the same point in 2022) (Office of New York Comptroller Brad Lander, 2023). Although bus ridership did not decrease to the same extent as subway ridership during the pandemic, it is recovering at a much slower rate, increasing only from 60% to 65% over the past year.

Tourism

New York had 66.6 million visitors in 2019, a tenth-consecutive annual record, generating $47.4 billion in spending. In 2020, pandemic travel restrictions caused a 67% reduction to 22.3 million, resulting in a loss of $1.2 billion in tax revenues (Office of the State Comptroller, 2021). In 2022, New York City hosted 56.7 million visitors, up from 32.9 million in 2021. In 2023, New York is expected to have more than 63 million visitors and to surpass 2019's record by 2024 (New York City Tourism & Conventions, 2023).

Unemployment

In early 2020, New York lost over one million jobs as the city became an epicenter of COVID-19. With only essential personnel working during lockdown, the city's record low unemployment rate of 3.7% shot up to 21% in May 2020 (Bhat & Welch, 2023). Currently, in 2023, New York's unemployment rate sits at 5.2%, approximately 40% above the national average of 3.6 % (New York Department of Labor, 2023).

Office Occupancy

According to the Office of the New York State Comptroller (2022), New York City's office sector employed a total of 1.6 million people in 2019, the highest level on record. Now, in 2023, New York City's vacant office space can fill 26.6 Empire State Buildings (Glaeser and Ratti). With the rise of remote and hybrid work, it is doubtful that the city's office occupancy rates will return to its pre-pandemic levels. A clear path forward has not yet materialized. The city is seeking to develop new sectors and to find alternative uses for these spaces. For example, rezoning efforts are now being considered to promote the possible conversion of office buildings into apartments (Schoifet, 2023). However, given the ever-widening gap between the rich and the poor in our global capital, it is likely that the push for luxury apartments by developers will most likely outweigh the need for affordable housing in Manhattan.

However, the future may shift because we are only now beginning the work of imagining New York's next chapter.

All of the above measures are still far from their pre-pandemic levels. According to the prepping practice of "situational awareness," these measures are far from their traditional baselines. One should, therefore, be cautious and develop a plan of action. New Yorkers should prepare to continue to "get comfortable in their discomfort" as the city's recovery is ongoing with probably more than one unexpected twist. For example, the successful transition to remote work suggests that New York's office sector will probably not return to the same capacity. Hirschman's 1970 options of *Exit, Voice, and Loyalty* come to mind. New Yorkers who remain anxious about the post-pandemic city may choose to move away or voice their concerns. Of course, loyalty to the city will affect one's decision to leave or push to have their voice heard.

I am loyal but I am fatigued. My best friend and I met recently over drinks to discuss the fate of New York. My best friend summarized this feeling best:

> As New Yorkers, all we do is respond and react to stuff now. I'm tired of it. I don't want to do it anymore. I am not like the preppers that you research. I am about the smooth mode, not the survival mode. Now, after the Union Square riot,[5] we have to worry about fighting kids, too? Really, it's too much.

Full disclosure: My best friend is emotionally scarred. Recently, she witnessed a subway rider perform fellatio on another passenger on the "A" train on a Wednesday afternoon ("The workday, Anna!"). According to her eye-witness report, one person had tarantula-like fake eyelashes; the other person wore a Kmart tracksuit. Musical accompaniment was provided via Boombox. My friend couldn't switch cars because she was on crutches. However, she did avert her eyes. Mostly.

Failing to prepare is preparing to fail. For preppers, emergency preparedness requires a careful review of previous disasters to determine how to better minimize risk to both person and property. Their review allows for the opportunity to test new strategies and tools for survival. In other words, preppers engage in processing and practicing new approaches to improve their resiliency. Sound advice for the city to avoid failing to prepare for the next pandemic was actually written by Daniel Defoe, the author of Robinson Crusoe (1719). *Due Preparations for the Plague, as Well as for Soul as Body* is a cross between a disaster response policy paper and a rudimentary guide for preppers, written to spur England (both its government and its subjects) to prepare to protect the country from an outbreak of the Bubonic Plague if it spread from Marseilles. In the book's introduction, Defoe (1722, p. 3) outlines the two key elements for preparing for a future pandemic; he calls for "Preparations *against* the Plague" and for "Preparations *for* the Plague." In preparing against the plague, the national and city governments are charged with enacting policies and plans to prevent the spread of the plague (such as restricting trade and enforcing quarantines). In preparations *for* the plague, individuals are responsible for "the personal and the particular" like gathering provisions and food for their families to shelter-in-place as well as limiting their travel and contact with outsiders. Over three hundred years later, Defoe's insight remains sound. Preparing *for* and preparing *against* a pandemic requires both government and citizens alike.

Given New York's position as an international gateway city, its elected leaders and public health officials should push to keep pandemic planning an agenda item for all levels of government. In an opinion piece in *The New York Times*, Dr. Tom Inglesby (2023), the director of the Johns Hopkins Center for Health Security and an expert in pandemic preparedness, argues that responding to a pandemic requires urgent and tough decisions that often have huge consequences for society. Public health leaders and policy makers must therefore be ready for such challenges in advance. He also notes, however, that Congress' "collective resolve to transform the country's pandemic response has diminished" (Inglesby, 2023). Key recommendations for strengthening a pandemic response include improving local public health capacity and better support for community organizations helping to alleviate the crisis (Inglesby, 2023).

City government also has a vital role to play in other recommendations, such as improving the distribution of tests and vaccines. New York seems poised to take on the challenge of developing a different set of tools and different levels of response to combat new pandemic threats. In late 2021, Mayor Bill de Blasio, the New York City Economic Development Corporation (NYCEDC), and the New York City Department of Health and Mental Hygiene (DOHMH) announced that Columbia University would launch and operate the Pandemic Response Institute (PRI), with its key partner, the CUNY Graduate School of Public Health and Health Policy (CUNY SPH) (Office of the Mayor, 2021). Working with diverse nonprofit organizations and community groups, the NYC PRI supports city agencies, organizations, and communities to prepare and respond to critical public health crises. As a comprehensive resource center, its main goals range from strengthening technologies to supporting real-time data collection and sharing, to centering racial equity in all activities to address gaps in the healthcare infrastructure (Office of the Mayor, 2021). To gain a better understanding of the complexity and all-encompassing tasks in planning a pandemic response for a global capital, one only needs to review the numerous missions and goals listed on the NYC PRI website.

A new public health plan for protecting the city against future pandemics may be in the offing, but there has been no real public dialog about needed changes. During the pandemic, dissatisfaction was certainly expressed.

However, public debate about pandemic prevention has never actually taken place. Instead, as a city, we just seem to keep moving forward. Moving *on* is not equivalent to moving *forward*. Since the pandemic officially ended in 2022, we have been moving on to the city's next chapter at the speed of a New York minute. Prior to the construction of the new World Trade Center, a public dialogue took place about the expectations and meaning of the new site as well as thinking about how we would honor those who were lost. Here is an example of the absence of public dialog. In May 2022, Mayor Eric Adams launched the NYC PRI, a new partnership with Columbia University and the City University of New York Graduate School of Public Health and Health Policy (CUNY SPH) to help New York City learn from the lessons of the COVID-19 pandemic and tackle the urgent public health emergencies currently facing New Yorkers – from infectious diseases to climate-related events (Office of the Mayor, 2022). However, the NYC PRI had been announced a year earlier by Mayor de Blasio (Office of the Mayor, 2021). There were no changes to the center's key partners nor to its mission. Did anyone notice this re-announcement? The announcements are nearly identical. However, in the second announcement, Mayor Adams states, "We can't wait for the next COVID-19 to arrive to look for downstream responses – we have urgent public health crises in our city, and we need to proactively face them with upstream solutions" (Office of the Mayor, 2022).[6] We can't wait? What?

Urban preppers can be invaluable local resources for information and support in preparing for and responding to disasters. Exploring their philosophy of preparedness and practices also provides valuable insight for disaster management and for preparing for the next pandemic. Furthermore, it has been argued that preppers and other community groups might be able to respond to some emergent needs at the local level; however, they cannot meet the needs of a larger population and wider region (Wright, 2022). That level of response typically requires a more complex network with key actors with stronger communication and distribution capabilities. Yet local resiliency sometimes exceeds expectations. Consider the impact of local resiliency in providing aid for Maui fire victims. In the Kahana community, Native Hawaiians coordinated an all-volunteer, large-scale disaster relief donation center that provided thousands of supplies brought in by an armada of private cruisers and catamarans from neighboring islands (Thebault, 2023). The effort had been organized independent of government as residents indicated that they had yet to receive aid from any agency (four days after the event). Local resiliency provides an immediate and effective stop-gap measure to aid residents. Resiliency depends not only on the power and resources of government but also on the efforts of citizens and community groups.

Two is One, One is None. As their use of prepper closets has demonstrated, preppers believe that having ample provisions are important during an emergency. This has been a tough lesson for many New Yorkers. Most people have had that experience of terror – being in a crowded place during the pandemic and losing a mask or having something happen to it and reaching into your pocket to discover that you did not bring an extra one. (Did you discover that you really cannot hold your breath as long as you imagined? I did.) That never happens to preppers. Usually, they are thinking about how the mask that they are wearing is suitable but that they should really test the new mask that they just read about.

Tragically, in New York, just like so many other places in the world, protective equipment and other essentials were in short supply during the pandemic. To prepare for the next pandemic, most experts argue that a stronger stockpile of equipment is needed. However, this recommendation may require revision. Both the national and state stockpiles proved inadequate for COVID-19. Given the lack of support from Republicans in Congress, the national stockpile was woefully underfunded and poorly maintained. New York State Governor Andrew Cuomo also jealously guarded the state stockpile. We didn't know much. We only knew that the city's healthcare workers and essential personnel lacked protective gear and that there were not enough ventilators.

In May 2020, the de Blasio administration began to create and maintain a 90-day stockpile of personal protective equipment (PPE) to better equip hospitals. During lockdown, the city also supplied over 7.5 million masks throughout the city as well as an additional 255,000 internet-enabled devices to students for remote learning (beyond the 175,000 devices that were provided at the start of the pandemic) (New York City Office of the Mayor, 2020).

As the federal government began to pit states against one another for supplies, an interesting possibility emerged as New York State, Delaware, and New Jersey began to work together to solve shortages. While this possibility did not move beyond preliminary talks, it did introduce regionalism as a strategy for responding to a pandemic.

In planning a route to leave the city, preppers do not rely only on what is in their bug-out bags, their own personal stockpile. Instead, they prepare to rely on a series of stockpiles. They often stash or bury caches filled with food and supplies along their designated route to use on the way to their final destination. These stockpiles are hidden in secret locations for their own use. However, they also sometimes work together to create and secure these stockpiles. They exchange information about these hidden caches so that they can support one another even if they are not traveling together. An important question in thinking about New York's future pandemic response would be to determine its approach to stockpiling. Should it continue to rely on an unreliable framework of national and state stockpiles with the expectation that it will create its own emergency stockpile if needed? Or should the city government, recognizing the unreliability of the national and state stockpiles, maintain its own stockpile and network with other cities or regions to maintain collective stockpiles?

Civilization is only three days of missed meals away from chaos.[7] This adage is a reminder about the importance of maintaining a food supply.[8] Preppers argue that hunger caused by a food shortage will lead to violence as people will begin fighting one another for food. The value of this adage came to mind when I received a call from a student and member of the military at the start of the pandemic. The young man was calling to tell me that his unit was now stationed at New Rochelle to provide provisions for those who had been quarantined. My student talked about the importance of providing food to residents, maintaining order and enforcing the boundaries of the quarantine. I recalled my sadness when I witnessed the Army troops arriving in my Greenwich Village neighborhood after the September 11 terrorist attacks in 2001. The troops arrived in our neighborhood to calm fears and to provide protection, if needed. As the caravan of green jeeps and trucks rumbled past me at Union Square Park, I was sad that it had come to this point. The last truck had a huge American flag draped over the back. The memory still brings tears to my eyes. I thought about the flag and our sense of citizenship and what binds us together. I was certainly grateful that the troops were there, but that moment made me realize the fragility of our lives and our misperceptions about safety. As he spoke, I thought about the scene in *Contagion* where people rush the Army truck for food. Our conversation about New Rochelle compounded my concern about the vulnerability of the city's food supply system. As the weeks passed, he would reach out to me again to share the heartbreak of loading bodies into 18-wheelers in the city.

The COVID-19 pandemic disrupted food availability and affordability and changed the daily food practices of New Yorkers in three critical ways: (1) the closing of restaurants and public institutions, including schools; (2) the economic disruption of reduced food access and changed shopping patterns, food expenditures, and diets; (3) the altered food practices and changed diets (Cohen, 2022). These harsh changes moved from abstraction to reality for me when I received a call from an old friend. Truth be told, I was surprised that she still had my number. She was no longer employed because her place of work, a restaurant, had shuttered. Like many New Yorkers, she had been standing in a long line to receive groceries at an emergency food pantry set up by the city government. The long lines were becoming overwhelming, and her fear was increasing. The family's food intake was insufficient and now very different from their usual diet of healthful meals. Now, her two children were both hungry and sick.

As with other hardships caused by the pandemic, the most vulnerable populations were disproportionately affected by these disruptions to New York's food system. While the city enacted emergency policies to combat food insecurity and hunger, the pandemic laid bare social equity issues within the city's food system. Post-pandemic, many social equity issues still exist, ranging from food deserts to disparities in access, to online grocers, to fears of participating in food assistance programs by immigrant groups.

The government is not your friend. The philosophy of self-reliance is rooted in the belief that the government will be unable or unwilling to help its citizens in an emergency situation. The response of all three levels of government confirmed this suspicion not just for preppers but for most Americans. Many Americans now share the sense that they cannot depend on government. For much of the 21st century, public trust in government has remained low. In 2022, only about two in ten Americans say they trust the government in Washington to do what is right "just about always" (2%) or "most of the time" (19%) (Pew Research Center, 2023). Furthermore, trust in the government has declined somewhat since 2021, when 24% reported that they could trust the government at least most of the time. For 2023, Gallup also recorded continued significant declines in public confidence in government institutions. With ratings within three points of their lowest all-time scores, few Americans feel a great deal of confidence about the presidency (26%), the Congress (8%), and the Supreme Court (27%) (Saad, 2023). Given President Donald Trump's mismanagement of the COVID-19 crisis, the loss of confidence in the federal government may, indeed, be warranted. However, policy failures occurred at all three levels of government, spurred by both political backbiting and competition among agencies at all levels.

Americans believe that increasing transparency, improving efficiency, and fixing leadership problems are key to increasing public trust in government (Pew Research Center, 2019). However, these changes cannot be made without a return to good government, which, according to Zakaria (2021, p. 53), involves "limited power but clear lines of authority. It is about giving officials autonomy, discretion, and the ability to exercise their own judgement." Recall the confusion caused by President Trump's micromanagement and lack of respect for Dr. Anthony Fauci and the Corona Virus Task Force. Central to the practice of good government is a renewed respect for and dedication to public service. While good government practices are needed at the federal and state levels, improving the resiliency of New York demands the application of good government at the local level. Significant investment (political, intellectual, and economic) and imagination will be required for this overhaul. A vital step in fostering good government is drawing lessons from how politics influence public health interventions and policies to prepare for the future, whether it is a resurgence of COVID-19 or the next pandemic. Important areas of investigation include examining social policy issues that promote public trust and compliance, both with pre-existing policies and those developed in response to COVID-19, and how the role of public institutions and the level of state capacity impact the control and delivery of healthcare services (Greer et al., 2020).

The Adams administration has not yet made such an investment. In his 2023 "State of the City" address, the mayor announced his "Working People's Agenda" that included a vast range of plans such as new job and workforce initiatives, anti-crime initiatives designed to reduce recidivism and gun violence, expanding tenant protections, free tax preparation programs, traffic safety improvements, additional public benefits, investments in public and green spaces, small business loans, student mental health programs, and universal dyslexia screenings. However, there was no mention of efforts to improve the quality of government or disaster preparedness. In November 2023, a federal criminal inquiry was initiated to determine if Mayor Adams's 2021 campaign conspired with the Turkish government and Turkish nationals to receive illegal donations (Rashbaum et al., 2023). A push for good government might begin with the installation of a new mayor.

The resiliency of New York depends on two elements – an engaged government and an engaged citizenry. This research reinforces that need for good government in planning for and responding to emergencies. Before the pandemic, preexisting conditions (like poverty) and the socially created vulnerabilities (such as overcrowded housing and unsafe working conditions during the pandemic) worked to make some populations even more vulnerable to COVID-19 (Wright, 2022). These dangers cannot be overcome by preparedness skills. Rather, the government should be held accountable to reduce these challenges and vulnerabilities through designing effective public policy. In this regard, vulnerability refers to "matters of power in that they reflect people's differential degrees of agency and their ability to affect change. Vulnerability suggests moral responsibilities for those in positions of power toward those who are less powerful" (Harrison, 2013, p. 110). However, policy changes to address vulnerabilities will not be made without the urging of an engaged citizenry. Alexis de Tocqueville's words remain true: "Among democratic nations all citizens are independent and weak; they can achieve almost nothing by themselves . . . therefore, they all sink into a state of impotence if they do not learn to help each other voluntarily."

In New York, the challenge is to restore the sense of possibility that could be gained by community and connection. In New York, the wide gap between the wealthy and those living in poverty is now enormous. According to the 2022 Census data, the wealthiest fifth of Manhattan residents earned an average income of $545,549, or more than 53 times as much as the bottom 20% who earned an average of $10,259 (Chen, 2023). This is the widest gap in the United States since 2006, when the data was first reported. An engaged urban citizenry is needed to plan a future with more hope than fear. However, we first need to find a way to bridge this gap to begin engaging with one another.

Notes

1 For an interesting revisit and rediscovery of Simmel's "The Metropolis and Mental Life" (1903), see Boy (2020).
2 New York has the worst urban heat island effects in comparison to any other major American city. According to a Climate Central study of 44 major U.S. cities, New York's concrete and steel skyscrapers and over 6,000 miles of asphalt absorb and radiate enough heat to make the city at least 8 degrees Fahrenheit hotter (Rosenberg, 2020).
3 See Jiménez et al. (2023) for a report on the blotting of the sun and wildfire smoke in Manhattan.
4 For an analysis of the great decline of crime in the United States, see Ford (2016).
5 Sparked by a social media influencer's promise to give away game consoles, the Union Square riot consisted of thousands of juveniles burning off energy as they battled with one another and the police. (Shanahan & Parnell, 2023). This incident may have the negative outcome of increasing the perception of juveniles as threats to public safety.
6 For a detailed analysis of Mayor Adam's rise to power, see Parker (2023).
7 This is actually a variation of Lenin's famous quotation: "Every society is three meals away from chaos."
8 For preppers, it is also a reminder about the Survival Rule of 3, which is critical knowledge for preparedness. According to the Survival Rule of 3 (backcountryliving.com): You can survive for 3 Minutes without air (oxygen) or in icy water; You can survive for 3 Hours without shelter in a harsh environment (unless in icy water); You can survive for 3 Days without water (if sheltered from a harsh environment); and You can survive for 3 Weeks without food (if you have water and shelter).

References

Akinnibi, F., & Wahid, R. (2022, July 29). Fear of rampant crime is derailing New York City's recovery. *Bloomberg*. www.bloomberg.com/graphics/2022-is-nyc-safe-crime-stat-reality/

Bhat, S., & Welch, W. (2023, August 5). How's New York City doing? Tracking our pandemic recovery. *The City*. https://projects.thecity.nyc/hows-new-york-city-doing/index.html

Boy, J. D. (2020). "The metropolis and the life of spirit" by Georg Simmel: A new translation. *The Journal of Classical Sociology*, *21*(2), 188–201. https://doi.org/10.1177/1468795X20980638

Chen, S. (2023, September 28). New York is rebounding for the rich. Nearly everyone else is struggling. *The New York Times*. www.nytimes.com/2023/09/28/nyregion/nyc-income-gap-wages.html

Closson, T., & Newman, A. (2022, January 15). Woman dies after being pushed onto subway tracks in Times Square. *The New York Times*. www.nytimes.com/2022/01/15/nyregion/woman-pushed-on-train-death.html

Cohen, N. (2022). Food crisis as a tool for social change: Lessons from New York City's COVID-19 response. *Urban Governance*, *2*(1), 173–177.

Fitzsimmons, E. G., & Root, J. (2023, July 31). Migrants will sleep outdoors because "there is no more room," Adams says. *The New York Times*. www.nytimes.com/2023/07/31/nyregion/migrants-sleeping-roosevelt-hotel.html

Ford, M. (2016, April 15). What caused the great crime decline in the U.S.? *The Atlantic*. www.theatlantic.com/politics/archive/2016/04/what-caused-the-crime-decline/477408/

Glaeser, E., & Ratti, C. (May 10, 2023). 26 Empire State Buildings could fit into New York's empty office space. That's a sign. *The New York Times*. https://www.nytimes.com/interactive/2023/05/10/opinion/nyc-office-vacancy-playground-city.html

Gordon, B. (2020). *Life after COVID-19: Lessons from past pandemics*. Banovallum Books.
Greer, S. L., King, E. J., da Fonseca, E. M., & Peralta-Santos, A. (2020). The comparative politics of COVID-19: The need to understand government responses. *Glob Public Health*, *15*(9), 1413–1416.
Harrison, E. (2013). Bouncing back? Recession, resilience and everyday lives. *Critical Social Policy*, *33*(1), 97–113
Inglesby, T. (2023, March 12). How to prepare for the next pandemic. *The New York Times*. www.nytimes.com/2023/03/12/opinion/pandemic-health-prepare.html
Jiménez, J., Bryson Taylor, D., & Jones, J. (2023, June 6). *Wildfire smoke blots sun and prompts health alerts in much of U.S.* https://www.nytimes.com/2023/06/06/us/canada-wildfires-us-smoke-air-quality.html
Maslin Nir, S., & Newman, A. (2022, April 12). Videos show an ordinary New York morning erupting into chaos on the N train. *The New York Times*. www.nytimes.com/2022/04/12/nyregion/video-brooklyn-shooting.html
Newman, A. (2023, June 28). A record 100,000 people in New York homeless shelters. *The New York Times*. www.nytimes.com/2023/06/28/nyregion/nyc-homeless-shelter-population.html
New York City Police Department. (2023, September 1). *NYPD citywide crime statistics August 2023*. www.nyc.gov/site/nypd/news/p00092/nypd-citywide-crime-statistics-august-2023
New York City Tourism & Conventions. (2023). *NYC travel & tourism outlook*. https://assets.ctfassets.net/1aemqu6a6t65/2Y8QEeyL0WPqNNSp2PF4tb/749947588ff25ed4bf119e6f9764420/2023_Travel_Tourism_Outlook_v3_f94a9a4a-c5dd-4a3d-bcfa-e5e13c2fe8d2.pdf
New York Health Foundation. (2023, June 21). Mental health of New Yorkers stagnates overall, worsens for some New Yorkers. *Press Release*. https://nyhealthfoundation.org/2023/06/21/mental-health-of-new-yorkers-stagnates-overall-worsens-for-some-new-yorkers/
New York State Department of Labor. (2023). *Current employment statistics*. https://dol.ny.gov/current-employment-statistics-0
Office of the Mayor. (2020, May 4). Test, trace & prepare: City creates stockpile of personal protective equipment. *Press Release*. www.nyc.gov/office-of-the-mayor/news/316-20/test-trace-prepare-city-creates-stockpile-personal-protective-equipment
Office of the Mayor. (2021, September 29). Mayor de Blasio announces Columbia University will operate and oversee pandemic response institute. *Press Release*. www.nyc.gov/office-of-the-mayor/news/660-21/mayor-de-blasio-columbia-university-will-operate-oversee-pandemic-response-institute
Office of the Mayor. (2022, May 12). Mayor Adams launches NYC pandemic response institute. *NYC.gov*. www.nyc.gov/office-of-the-mayor/news/287-22/mayor-adams-launches-nyc-pandemic-response-institute
Office of New York Comptroller Brad Lander. (2023, March 16). *Riders return: As New Yorkers return to buses and subways, some pandemic ridership trends are here to stay*. https://comptroller.nyc.gov/reports/riders-return/
Office of the New York State Comptroller. (2022). *The office sector in New York City*. www.osc.state.ny.us/files/reports/osdc/pdf/report-11-2022.pdf
Parker, I. (2023, August 7). Eric Adams' administration of bluster. *The New Yorker*. www.newyorker.com/magazine/2023/08/14/eric-adams-profile
Pew Research Center. (2019, July 22). *Americans' solutions for trust-related problems*. www.pewresearch.org/politics/2019/07/22/americans-solutions-for-trust-related-problems/
Pew Research Center. (2023, September 19). *Public Trust in Government: 1958–2023*. www.pewresearch.org/politics/2023/09/19/public-trust-in-government-1958-2023/

Pozarycki, R. (2022, October 24). Crunching the numbers: Yes, crime is up – but NYC is still safer than it was two decades ago. The NYPD's statistics prove it. *AMNY*. www.amny.com/news/crime-up-nyc-still-safer/
Quinnipiac University Poll. (2022, May 4). Crime overshadows all other issues as the most urgent in NYC, Quinnipiac University New York City poll finds; but half of voters say they expect tourism to increase. *Press Release*. https://poll.qu.edu/images/polling/nyc/nyc05042022_nydg85.pdf
Rashbaum, W. K., Rubinstein, D., & Rothfeld, M. (2023, November 10). F.B.I. seizes Eric Adams's phones as campaign investigation intensifies. *The New York Times*. www.nytimes.com/2023/11/10/nyregion/adams-fbi-investigation-phones.html#:~:text=F.B.I.%20agents%20seized%20Mayor%20Eric,funnel%20money%20into%20its%20coffers
Rosenberg, J. (2020, August 13). New York City has America's greatest heat islands. By great we mean the worst. *Gothamist*. https://gothamist.com/news/new-york-city-has-americas-greatest-heat-islands-by-great-we-mean-the-worst
Routhier, G. (2019). State of the homeless 2019. *Coalition for the Homeless*. www.coalitionforthehomeless.org/state-of-the-homeless-2019
Ryan, C. (2015). Everyday resilience as resistance: Palestinian women practicing sumud. *International Political Sociology*, *9*(4), 299–315.
Saad, L. (2023, July 6). *Historically low faith in U.S. institutions continues*. https://news.gallup.com/poll/508169/historically-low-faith-institutions-continues.aspx
Schimmenti, A., Billieux, J., & Starcevic, V. (2020). The four horsemen of fear: An integrated model of understanding fear experiences during the COVID-19 pandemic. *Clinical Neuropsychiatry: Journal of Treatment Evaluation*, *17*(2), 41–45.
Schoifet, M. (2023, August 17). NYC kicks off plan to rezone Midtown, turn offices to houses. *Bloomberg*. www.msn.com/en-us/money/realestate/nyc-kicks-off-plan-to-rezone-midtown-turn-offices-into-housing
Shanahan, E., & Parnell, W. (2023, August 4). YouTube streamer faces riot charge after Union Square Park erupts in chaos. *The New York Times*. www.nytimes.com/2023/08/04/nyregion/union-square-kai-cenat-twitch-giveaway.html
Simmel, G. (1903). *The metropolis and mental life*. Blackwell Publishing.
Southall, A., & Schweber, N. (2022, May 24). Man fatally shot on Manhattan subway in unprovoked attack. *The New York Times*. www.nytimes.com/2022/05/22/nyregion/nyc-subway-shooting.html
Survivalist Prepper. (n.d.). *Situational awareness: what it means to be preppers*. Retrieved August 6, 2023, from https://survivalistprepper.net/situational-awareness-what-it-means-to-preppers/
Thebault, R. (2023, August 12). Native Hawaiians organize aid for Maui fire victims as government lags. *The Washington Post*. www.washingtonpost.com/nation/2023/08/12/maui-fires-lahaina-native-hawaiians-disaster-relief-boats/
Wright, K. (2022). *Community resilience: A critical approach*. Routledge.
Zakaria, F. (2021). *Ten lessons for a post-pandemic world* (Norton paperback ed.). W.W. Norton & Company.

8

RESILIENCY AND A WAY FORWARD FOR THE CITY

My first book on New York City's preppers closed with my thanking this community for teaching me how to pack a bug-out bag. Thanks to urban preppers, I already had an N-95 mask at the outset of the pandemic. I will be forever grateful for their willingness to share their knowledge. However, I must confess that these preppers didn't teach me everything about sheltering in place. Provided below is an entry from my journal written in early June 2020. I still agree with it.

Things that NYC Preppers Should Have Taught Me

Now that COVID-19 has not just disappeared or vaporized in the summer heat (as promised by Trump), it is time to think about how to improve my survival game for the rest of the year. Sure, attending virtual meetings and watching those city prepper YouTube clips taught me some additional lessons about sheltering in place during lockdown; however, I also now realize that preppers may be withholding critical knowledge on survival in the city. Knowing how to make your own hand sanitizer or sourdough starter is great, but they missed a few important tips.

Chip Clips should be stockpiled. Based on my lack of Chip Clips, too many open bags of chips have become a dangerous force in my home by blocking any chance of counter-space productivity (not to mention weight loss). They have formed a teetering Tower of Chipza in my kitchen. In keeping with the urban prepper ethos of ingenuity, I have been using the stern Jumbo Office Binder Clips that normally hold together stacks of boring documents that no one ever reads. They serve their purpose, but these gigantic clips are too judgmental. I miss the friendly nature of the Chip Clip. There are actually two

DOI: 10.4324/9781003400356-8

types of Chip Clips, each welcoming in its own way. The streamlined Chip Clip reassures you that you look great (even better than before you started sheltering in place). The clip is thin; therefore, *you* are thin. The second type of Chip Clip is usually blessed with a cute animal face that encourages snacking. The snap of the friendly raccoon Chip Clip promises more fun later by saying, "Don't worry, the chips love you, too. Come back whenever you'd like. And, it's OK, if it's just two minutes from now." Conversely, the Jumbo Office Binder Clip clamps shut with a brutal finality that says, "We're closing up shop. Indefinitely. You've had enough. Maybe I am not the jumbo one." This alienation has led even to the early demise of a bag of Popchips due to my social distancing from the rude Binder Clip.

Favorite pastimes of family members cannot be denied no matter how loathsome. Bringing out new games and entertainment to boost family morale is useless. Netflix, board games, books, cards, and crafts will never top my spouse's favorite pastimes. Nothing beats the nostalgia of playing the "Remember That Time?" game, which begins out of nowhere and usually when you are not feeling like your normal champion self. While not actually a contact sport, this game does demand an instant "flight or fight" response. Play with caution as opponents can be wounded. The game always starts with a swift round of something like "Remember that time you booked a spa weekend with your friends on my birthday?" [I only considered it before I realized the date.] You know the sort of fun that I'm talking about. Watch out for rabbit punches like: "Remember that time you insisted on wearing new flip flops and walked slowly to make us late for the new *Stars Wars* movie?" [They were new wedges. I had a blister. We also arrived 30 minutes early. Early.] To end the game, I usually bust out a legendary haymaker like, "Remember that time you insisted that we go to your parents' home for Thanksgiving and promised that we would celebrate with my family the following year but my parents divorced before the next Thanksgiving? I certainly do." Well, I wanted to win, right?

Highlighting and coloring are survival skills. I am not referring to glossing over the pain of sloughing through emails that I should have replied to well before the pandemic and highlighting only my workday achievements such as scoring a good deal from "Wirecutter" on barbeque tongs for a grill that I do not own. I am also not talking about my ability to tell a colorful story or joke (I am a sailor's kid). My pre-COVID life was more colorful than the New York Botanical Gardens on the finest spring day. All joy. However, after one month at home, I am obsessed only with one color – that pasty oatmeal-ish color that is usually found in the diaper of a newborn. Without the magic touch of a colorist, that's the shade that New York Blonde becomes without care. New York City Preppers did not warn me about this. Surely, I should be able to paint some essential oil on my hair to solve this problem. I just need to know how long I need to wrap up the painted hair strips in aluminum foil. Colorists should be considered essential workers. I have tried everything from shampoos to dye to voodoo. I've settled on a custom color of my own design, Hamster Blonde. A primer on giving your partner a haircut that does not make him look like a member of the Peeky Blinders Gang would be great, too.

You can't stockpile the divine. Before the pandemic, I sometimes stopped by my church, St. Francis Xavier, to light a candle and pray. In those moments of solitude and prayer, I could feel God's grace. Sure, a homeless person would sometimes get rowdy and ruin the vibe. However, that rarely happened. I stopped going to Mass years ago. The church has a formal name for lapsed Catholics like me – "Runaways." Why did I stop going? The loss of too many loved ones, I think. At five bucks a candle, it adds up. No, it wasn't the money. It was the heartache that was costing me too much; or, maybe it was being shocked by a reporter who stopped me on the church steps after Mass one Sunday to ask my feelings about the pedophilia practiced by men who were supposed to be leaders of my faith. The disgust of that reality definitely made me turn away. Yet, during lockdown, I find myself longing for the strength that one finds in worshipping as a part of a community. I keep thinking about all of us huddled together in our church on September 11 and 12, singing and praying together. Lately, when I meditate, I feel a spark of the divine. Faith and grace are not items that you can store on a shelf to use whenever you need them. Like prepping skills, they demand dedicated practice.

Clearly, one can argue that this journal entry reveals my subject position. The ability to have such minor concerns reflects the privilege of affluence. That's true. However, I think my reflections also reveal something more significant. They demonstrate the power of the pandemic to affect every aspect of our lives, to unmoor us by whittling away at all things from the mundane to the sacred. Every single thing.

My journal entry also reveals the significance of the lessons that the preppers didn't teach me. The preppers weren't able to teach me very much about how to negotiate the realities of life that existed before, during, and after the pandemic, like our spiritual and emotional needs, our ordinary relationship challenges, our symbolic interpretations of our surroundings, as well as our personal identities. That's the business of living, not just surviving. Therefore, this chapter first discusses NYC prepping practices as possible local resiliency strategies, focusing on preparedness, adaptation, and community. This chapter also outlines the core components needed for strengthening the city's resiliency, purpose, evolution, and community-building.

Researching and sharing the experience of New Yorkers during the pandemic has been a challenging process. Throughout this project, my goal has been to practice my own form of resiliency as a researcher. Research resilience is defined as "the ability to adapt and continue the research throughout a crisis while maintaining consistency with the overall research design to successfully complete a research project" (Rahman et al., 2021, p. 3). My resiliency approach has been two-pronged. I have carried out the study in a stable and reliable manner throughout the pandemic, and I have attempted to do more than just endure the pandemic, remaining productive in conducting my research (Vargo & Seville, 2011). It is also important to note that continuing my research during the pandemic may have been easier for me, given my research focus on a subculture that trains in emergency preparedness and community resilience literature.

In my first book about urban preppers, I discussed how studying the rise of prepping in New York had enriched my understanding of urbanism by "finding new problems that I hadn't imagined, new aspects of that world I haven't imagined, new ways of thinking about phenomena of everyday life wherever it occurs" (Lu, 2015, p. 128). The identity of an urban prepper – a city dweller who prepares and trains to protect his or her family against disaster – is a sharp contrast to the classic depictions of an urbanite characterized by a blasé attitude and indifference (Simmel, 1903) or by adhering to an etiquette of reservation and formality to serve as a buffer in a city of strangers (Sennett, 1992). To my surprise, NYC preppers were combining their knowledge of city life with knowledge about homesteading and bushcraft skills. I argued that, at least for some New Yorkers, prepping may reflect a new city sensibility. With the perception of increased risk and public anxiety about governmental and economic instability, environmental catastrophic, pandemic, and technological collapse (Beck, 2009), some New Yorkers felt that city life demanded "street smarts" and "survival smarts." In a recent interview with Bradley Garrett on his podcast, "Tenacity," I suggested that this new sensibility may be an emerging structure of feeling (Williams, 1977). As we discussed Garrett's questions about prepping in the city, I talked about how preparedness is becoming a part of New York culture. While New Yorkers are preparing for disaster on different levels and in different ways, our conversation was rooted in the reality of real New Yorkers trying to protect their families by practicing self-reliance and by relying on the power of community.

Now that we all have experienced the COVID-19 pandemic, the stigma against preppers seems to be declining. As I explained in my first book, when people discovered my research subject, some individuals would try to nudge me into stating that preppers are crazy people who are obsessed by conspiracy theories. When I refused to confirm their suspicions by making that broad claim, I could sometimes actually see their perception of me shift – a raised eyebrow, an almost imperceptible nod of (mis)understanding, or the faint trace of a smirk. Their expressions were sometimes signs of a false sense of superiority because I had clearly "gone native." Later I came to recognize negative comments as responses to fear. A sincere conversation about the possibility of disaster and measures to protect against harm is a disturbing subject. This time around, people do not shy away from talking with me. Instead, they reach out to me to talk over their plans and concerns. At the start of the pandemic, I received a phone call from a colleague. She called to let me know that she was disappointed that I didn't hold a Zoom meeting to share my knowledge with my department. She argued that I had a responsibility to try to help people. No doubt, there has been a change in the perception of preppers.

Throughout the pandemic, I have tried to focus on the request made by a prepper at the start of my research. Annette, a skilled prepper of several years as well as a mother and wife, asked me to make sure that readers understand that preppers are not preparing for the end of the world. Rather, as she explained to me, "We are preparing for tomorrow. Tomorrow." I often turn that phrase over in my mind. Some days it feels like an inspirational quote that I should be posting on Instagram. It reminds me of the most important lessons that my time with urban preppers have taught me about self-reliance: preparedness, adaptation, and community. The federal government's mishandling of the pandemic response has destroyed the bond between the nation state and its citizens. Becoming self-reliant and being prepared for disaster are critical to protecting one's family in the absence of government aid. NYC preppers demonstrated the effectiveness of preparedness strategies such as maintaining a prepper closet that is stocked with emergency food, provisions, and medical supplies. Having emergency savings ("go money") also helped preppers who experienced job loss and economic hardship during the pandemic. Adaptation, "getting comfortable in your discomfort," was also useful to preppers in adjusting to the new challenges of life while sheltering-in-place. As they were already prepared for the possibility of a pandemic, NYC preppers bolstered their neighborhoods and communities through actions such as serving as information resources to help non-preppers to plan for the pandemic and by utilizing their rich resource networks to secure (and sometimes even deliver) needed supplies. In addition, urban preppers met online to troubleshoot the practical challenges of sheltering-in-place and to exchange notes about the safety of different areas of the city. Preppers also talked with one another to provide support and encouragement during the loss of loved ones and the loss of employment. All of these activities worked to increase community resilience during the COVID-19 pandemic lockdown.

To fully understand the potential of the urban prepping community as a model of local resilience, further investigation must be completed. After Hamas's October 7 attack on Israel, Inshirah, the founder of a woman's prepping group and a former leader of the NYCPN, reached out to me and explained that she wanted to have a meeting of female preppers to work through ideas because, "as women and as mothers, we are responsible for protecting our children and we need to devise plans for their safety." Inshirah's comment is powerful because it signals a continued belief in self-reliance and the perception that, given their role as caregivers, female preppers may have a different approach to preparedness. In the weeks before the pandemic, I began working on a new project designed to study the motivations and practices of female preppers. My project aims to analyze the perspectives of American female preppers as their survival strategies are often rooted in caretaking, homesteading, and sustainability practices. I now plan to return to this project seeking to explore how gender may influence the practice of preparedness and prepping culture. In a *New York Times* op-ed piece, Mira Ptacin, a homemaker-turned-prepper during the pandemic, acknowledged that the female understanding of preparedness may be rooted more in family tradition than fear of the apocalypse. According to Ptacin (2020 para. 11),

> instead of embracing my inner Mad Max, I could channel my own mother and grandmother, and a bit of Survival Mom – to be a nurturing, resourceful and resilient homemaker ready for anything. If Mad Max is the yang of prep – the masculine, overt energy – then I wanted to tap into the yin of prep, the earthy, feminine energy. The yin of prep is about extending your network of neighbors and friends to build resilience in your household, your neighborhood and your community.

My research involves interviewing and learning from female prepping experts, independent female preppers, leaders, and members of all female prepping groups as well as female leaders of mixed groups. I hope to discover if and how their approach is different from male preppers. Although I have only just returned to this project, it seems topics such as homesteading, personal safety, women's health, reproduction, and prepping with children should be emphasized.

A series of comparative analyses of the prepper subcultures of global capitals should also be conducted to determine how each city's unique elements such as risk, culture, economy, and geography shape these groups and their local resilience strategies. For example, given the pandemic and fear about the rise in natural disasters, interest in prepping and the investment in prepping supplies have grown across the UK (Ambrose, 2023). A comparison between New York and London prepping groups would provide insight into how a city's characteristics inform approaches to disaster preparedness.

At the start of sheltering in place, I made silly resolutions just like I do on New Year's Eve – I am going to work out every day right after I jot down some beautiful prose in my gratitude journal. You probably made a few silly resolutions, too. (You can always share them with me in a text or email. I won't tell anyone.) However, I am not talking about committing to that nonsense. Instead, I am talking about the real promises that I made in my secret heart about loving people better when I thought that the world might end. I committed to something better. Maybe you did, too. I had forgotten those promises until I was nearly done with this book. In reviewing the work of NYC preppers and so many other people during the pandemic, I am again reminded of Emerson's words: "Character teaches above our wills."

As a Queens college professor who has witnessed the impact of COVD-19 on my students, I now believe college plans and programs that are designed to aid students during a disaster should be studied as strategies of local resilience. In examining the impact of the COVID-19 pandemic on college students' health and financial stability in New York, a survey of CUNY students (Jones et al., 2021) found that over half (54.5%) of students reported anxiety/depression, with 49% reporting increased need for mental health services. The majority of students (81.1%) reported a loss of household income, with half (49.8%) reporting worries about losing housing. High levels of food and housing insecurity were also found. Food insecurity, depression and anxiety are all significant risks because they serve as a barrier to academic achievement (Silva et al., 2015; Eisenberg et al., 2009). In turn, these risks jeopardize the likelihood of graduating from college, an important key in achieving economic success. From attending class to participating in clubs or sports to enjoying time with friends, the college experience provides stability and security for students. I am thinking about our college's immediate local acts of resilience to support one another during lockdown. For example, the Knights Table Food Pantry created an innovative way to provide food to Queens College students and their families. Since students could not visit the pantry on campus, the Knights Table delivered groceries to students and their families in designated neighborhoods. As announced on the college's website and on social media, students just had to sign up and pick up groceries from the Knights Table delivery truck. I remain moved by this service because it represents the dignity and sense of humanity that we try to instill in our students. Our college's motto is *Discimus ut serviamus*: We learn so that we may serve. After helping my students endure the loss of loved ones and the hardships of job loss, the pandemic has taught me that working to strengthen student resiliency in all of its forms, from providing a lecture to providing a meal, is a fundamental act of teaching and service.

So, as a New Yorker, as a researcher, and as a teacher, what does committing to something better mean? For me, it means committing to the resiliency of the city. For the last two semesters, I have taught a writing-intensive course in which my students and I examine the problems and possibilities of post-pandemic New York. We study the potential viability of programs designed to strengthen the city's recovery. Their research projects have ranged from a New York Climate Corps to enrichment programs for the children in our public elementary schools who fell behind during the pandemic to inventive support programs for small businesses owned by People of Color. After studying the effects of the 1918 influenza pandemic on New York, one of my students raised an important question, and a revelation for me. The college senior commented:

> In our class, we've learned so many things about this pandemic. We've got ideas to share. What about our understanding of our experience with COVID-19? If we are lucky, maybe there won't be another pandemic for a hundred years. But that means none of us is going to be around. We won't be alive. We won't be there to share our firsthand knowledge and our personal experiences. It's all going to be lost.

Our class grew quiet as everyone contemplated this sad reality. After a few moments, someone cracked a smile and said, "Séance. They can reach us by séance." We all laughed. In response to her question, I talked about how people were going to learn about this pandemic just like we have learned about other pandemics. They would learn through studying archival research, like news reports, first-person accounts and by reading scholarship on COVID-19. She didn't seem satisfied. She shook her head in protest and replied, "There won't be 'us.' There won't be people living with actual memories. We will all be gone. The idea of a pandemic won't be real anymore."

Her concern has stayed with me. It seems that there are two issues. Given the closeness of the world, I fear that another pandemic will not wait for a hundred years. Second, her concern also seems to be a call to action. After living through such a tumultuous experience, how does one not just move forward, but how does one try to transform the experience of surviving the pandemic into a sign of hope for the future?

Studying the lived experience of New York preppers and others who stayed in the city during lockdown has provided critical insight into understanding local preparation for and response to disaster. My research suggests that preparedness, adaptation, and community are key elements to local resiliency. However, these principles are not all useful to envisioning New York's future. Preparedness for the city's future is more than planning for the next disaster and improving our disaster response. Our purpose is even bolder. Instead, as urban citizens, a clear agenda is needed for New York. That's what a positive future requires of us. Endurance. Work. For preppers, adaptation seems to be grounded in the stoic's perception of focusing on limitation and adjustment. Instead, we must commit, not just to surviving, but committing to something better. The federal government's mismanagement of the pandemic exposed the instability of our democracy. Rather than adapting to the government's inadequacies, we should evolve by demanding that the needs of citizens be met by government rather than relinquishing this expectation (Haas, 2023). This objective cannot be met without strengthening our connections with one another.

As the psychiatrist Robert Lifton (2023, p. xxviii) argues, "the survivor suffers from catastrophe but can also be crucial to overcoming it. By looking closely at the struggles of survivors, we can learn much about the catastrophe itself and about the larger human capacity for collective renewal." Imagine the possibilities for our city if public discourse on recovery focused on the principles of purpose, evolution, and community-building. If we cut away the rhetoric behind the importance of being a global capital, what would be the meaningful purpose of the city? What do we fight for? What do we fight against? How do we define community? Now when I think about the exodus of the rich from the city at the start of the pandemic, I spend more time thinking about the millions who stayed behind. We held together, and we continued to function as a city. What held us together? It was the belief in the city and in one another that was important. Lifton argues:

> Survivors – whether of wars, nuclear explosions, the ongoing climate emergency, Covid, or other catastrophic events – can lead others on a path to reinvention. If human life is unsustainable as we have become accustomed to living it, it is likely up to survivors – people who have stared into the abyss of catastrophe – to imagine and enact new ways of living.
>
> *(Gessen, 2023, para 6)*

Therefore, we must develop a deeper understanding of New York's resiliency, contemplating new ways of living. Surprisingly, a historic Manhattan neighborhood may provide a fresh way of thinking about the city's future and the power of local resiliency. A preliminary review suggests that Stuyvesant Town is one potential example of local resilience that seeks to protect its residents on many fronts: affordability, sustainability, and disaster response. Originally built for World War II veterans and their families, Stuyvesant Town – Peter Cooper Village – is a large post–World War II residential development on Manhattan's East Side. Built on 80 acres that now contains abundant green space, Stuyvesant Town contains 11,250 apartments. It is best known for its middle-class residents' struggle to save their homes against real estate giants (Garodnick, 2021). Beyond maintaining affordable housing, Stuyvesant Town has also worked to improve its sustainability by installing energy-efficient technology such as solar panels and LED lighting systems (Stuytown.com, n.d.a). Stuyvesant Town has installed urban farming pods throughout the 80-acre neighborhood in 2022 (Stuytown.com, n.d.b). The pods now produce over two tons of vegetables annually. The produce is distributed to elderly and disabled residents of the neighborhood as well as to those in need across the city. Stuyvesant also added 10 beehives to neighborhood rooftops to help pollinate local flora. Many residents also participate in a community gifting program designed to save money and to reduce waste. Sports, exercise and self-defense classes are also available to residents. A small, free library is available for adults and children. During the pandemic, a community network was formed to ensure that the elderly and disabled received deliveries of food and medicine.

Central to its success seems to be robust civic engagement and community dialogue. Stuyvesant's resiliency is supported by its active tenant association that monitors policies implemented by property management and advocates for the interests of residents. In turn, neighborhood critics of the tenant association also post periodic blogs to report the association's perceived shortcomings. In addition, community members also debate issues on various Facebook pages dedicated to the neighborhood. Neighbors also gather in parochial spaces to discuss their viewpoints. The Stuyvesant Town model has a system of public administration offices, representative organizations, and an executive branch as well as public discussion forums. While imperfect, Stuyvesant may represent the democratic spirit as expressed by De Tocqueville.

Traditionally, a book's last chapter presents study conclusions and future directions for research. In reviewing my chapter, it seems that I have also created a plan for my life's work – a mission of sorts – committing to the resiliency of the city and placing my faith in the local. On a recent day, I had just returned from a walk across the East Village. I had been thinking about the fate of the city. On Instagram, Jason, the leader of the NYCPN, had posted about how the retirement of 250 NYC police officers means a likely increase in crime for the city. His next post entailed puzzling through the mystery of the new White Lung variant. Jason is always complaining about the city, yet he is always trying to save all 8.8 million of us. He can't always be thinking that the city is that bad, though. I shot him a text to pose that very question. What does he love about the city? For him, it's the excellent choice of restaurants and its accessibility. See? He isn't always thinking about the apocalypse. He sometimes thinks about food and how fast he can get to it. I paused for a moment outside my apartment building. When I looked up from my phone, I discovered that the sunlight of the golden hour had hit the bricks of my apartment building just right. For a moment, my boring apartment building was set ablaze in a gorgeous color storm of red and orange hues. I recalled that my friend, Suzanne, had shared that her grandfather, David J. Strickland, created and manufactured those bricks. I thought about his artistry in creating that special color. All of those years ago, he was adding to the resilience and glory of the city. It is our turn now.

I am closing on joy. Join me.

References

Ambrose, T. (2023, November 11). "People are worried": The "prepper" shops serving Britons who fear doomsday is coming. *The Guardian*. www.theguardian.com/business/2023/nov/11/people-are-worried-the-prepper-shops-serving-britons-who-fear-doomsday-is-coming

Beck, U. (2009). *World at risk*. Polity Press.
Eisenberg, D., Golberstein, E., & Hunt, J. B. (2009). Mental health and academic success in college. *The B.E. Journal of Economic Analysis & Policy*, *9*, 40.
Garodnick, D. R. (2021). *Saving Stuyvesant town: How one community defeated the worst real estate deal in history*. Cornell University Press.
Gessen, M. (2023, November 12). How to maintain hope in an age of catastrophe. *The New Yorker*. www.newyorker.com/news/the-new-yorker-interview/how-to-maintain-hope-in-an-age-of-catastrophe
Haas, M. (2023). *Beyond polarized American democracy: From mass society to coups and civil war*. Taylor & Francis.
Jones, H. E., Manze, M., Ngo, V., Lamberson. P., & Freudenberg, N. (2021). The impact of the COVID-19 pandemic on college students' health and financial stability in New York City: Findings from a population-based sample of City University of New York (CUNY) students. *Journal of Urban Health*, *98*, 187–196.
Lifton, R. J. (2023). *Surviving our catastrophes: Resilience and renewal from Hiroshima to the COVID-19 pandemic*. The New Press.
Lu, W. (2015). Sociology and art: An interview with Howard S. Becker. *Symbolic Interaction*, *38*(1), 127–150.
Ptacin, M. (2020, September 24). I am not a housewife, I'm a prepper. *The New York Times*. www.nytimes.com/2020/09/24/opinion/sunday/i-am-not-a-housewife-im-a-prepper.html
Rahman, S. A., Tuckerman, L., Vorley, T., & Gherhes, C. (2021). Resilient research in the field: Insights and lessons from adapting qualitative research projects during the COVID-19 pandemic. *International Journal of Qualitative Methods*, *20*, 1–16.
Sennett, R. (1992). *The uses of disorder: Personal identity & city life* (2nd ed.). Vintage Books.
Silva, M. R., Kleinert, W. L., Sheppard, A. V., Cantrell, K. A., Freeman-Coppadge, D. J., Tsoy, E., Roberts, T., & Pearrow, M. (2015). The relationship between food security, housing stability, and school performance among college students in an urban university. *Journal of College Student Retention: Research, Theory & Practice*, *19*(3), 284–299.
Simmel, G. (1903). *The metropolis and mental life*. Blackwell Publishing.
Stuytown. (n.d.a). *Powering forward: Our sustainability journey*. www.stuytown.com/sustainability
Stuytown. (n.d.b). *Stuytown welcomes urban farming by MicroHabitat*. www.stuytown.com/microhabitat
Vargo, J., & Seville, E. (2011). Crisis strategic planning for SMEs: Finding the silver lining. *International Journal of Production Research*, *49*(18), 5619–5635.
Williams, R. (1977). *Marxism and literature*. Oxford University Press.

INDEX

Note: Page numbers in italics indicate a figure and page numbers in bold indicate a table on the corresponding page.